Mahdi Asghari Ozma
Amin Abbasi
Hossein Samadi Kafil

Postbiotics in Medical Bacteriology

nova
Medicine & Health
New York

DOI: https://doi.org/10.52305/UTVW6627

Library of Congress Cataloging-in-Publication Data

ISBN: 979-8-89530-559-1 (Softcover)
ISBN: 979-8-89530-652-9 (eBook)

Published by Nova Science Publishers, Inc. † New York

"Postbiotics are one of the most exciting areas of research in modern microbiology, and Postbiotics in Medical Bacteriology provides an outstanding and comprehensive look at this rapidly growing field. This book not only elucidates the complex mechanisms through which postbiotics exert their effects but also presents their practical applications in medicine, offering a clear roadmap for their therapeutic potential. The authors have successfully synthesized cutting-edge research, clinical insights, and real-world applications, making this work an invaluable resource for researchers, clinicians, and anyone interested in the evolving role of microbiota in health and disease."

— Dr. Anahita Ghorbani Tajani, PhD,
University of Wyoming, Laramie, USA

"This book is an essential read for those interested in advancing our understanding of the role of postbiotics in human health. With a strong foundation in medical bacteriology, it skillfully covers the complexities of probiotics, prebiotics, and synbiotics, while providing a detailed exploration of postbiotics as a therapeutic tool. The authors' ability to present complex scientific concepts in a clear and accessible manner will make this book a valuable asset for both academic researchers and practitioners in the field."

— Dr. Sahar Sabahi, PhD,
Director of Nutrition Department
Ahvaz University of Medical Sciences, Ahvaz, Iran

This book is dedicated to the countless researchers, scientists, and healthcare professionals who continue to push the boundaries of knowledge in the field of microbiome science, particularly in the study of probiotics, prebiotics, synbiotics, and postbiotics. Their dedication to improving human health and well-being through microbiota modulation and therapeutic interventions serves as the foundation of this work.

We also dedicate this book to our families, whose unwavering support and encouragement have been invaluable throughout the writing process. Their understanding, patience, and belief in the importance of this research have provided us with the strength to continue, even in the most challenging times.

Lastly, this book is dedicated to the future of science—those researchers, students, and innovators who will build upon these concepts and continue to discover new ways to enhance human health and treatment paradigms. May this work serve as a small step in a much larger journey toward a healthier and more sustainable world for all.

Contents

Foreword

The study of the human microbiome has experienced an extraordinary transformation over the past few decades. From its early recognition as a critical element of digestion to its emerging role in influencing a wide array of health conditions, the microbiome has become central to our understanding of human health. In particular, research on probiotics, prebiotics, synbiotics, and postbiotics has illuminated the profound impact of microorganisms and their metabolic products on our physiological and immune systems.

One of the most intriguing and rapidly developing areas of this field is postbiotics—the non-viable microbial products or byproducts that exert beneficial health effects. Postbiotics have the potential to revolutionize therapeutic approaches by offering a stable, safe, and effective alternative to live probiotics. Unlike live probiotics, which face challenges in survival and efficacy under diverse conditions, postbiotics can offer the same, if not more, therapeutic benefits without the risks of microbial translocation or infection.

In Postbiotics in Medical Bacteriology, the authors, Dr. Mahdi Asghari Ozma, Dr. Amin Abbasi, and Dr. Hossein Samadi Kafil, have compiled a comprehensive and forward-thinking resource on the use of postbiotics in medicine. This book offers not only a thorough overview of the scientific principles behind postbiotics, but also a practical exploration of their applications in medical treatment. The work provides an invaluable resource for both researchers and clinicians seeking to understand the mechanisms through which postbiotics exert their effects, and the potential therapeutic applications they offer.

The chapters in this book span a wide range of topics, from the fundamental concepts of probiotics, prebiotics, and synbiotics to an in-depth examination of the bioactive components of postbiotics and their safety assessments. The authors meticulously explore the preparation techniques, regulatory considerations, and the bio-utilization of postbiotics in treating gastrointestinal, metabolic, and immune-related disorders. With a particular emphasis on postbiotics' potential role in reducing inflammation, improving gut health, and enhancing metabolic function, this book paves the way for future therapeutic innovations. What sets this book apart is the authors' ability to bridge the gap between basic microbiological research and its clinical applications. By combining cutting-edge scientific discoveries with practical insights, they have created a work that is both informative and accessible, providing readers with the knowledge they need to harness the potential of postbiotics in the real world.

I have no doubt that this book will inspire further research, ignite new ideas, and, ultimately, contribute to the advancement of microbiome-based therapies that will improve the health and well-being of individuals around the world.

Professor Hedayat Hosseini, PhD, DVM
Shahid Beheshti University of Medical Sciences
Tehran, Iran

Acknowledgments

We would like to express our deepest gratitude to all those who have supported and contributed to the completion of this book, Postbiotics in Medical Bacteriology. This project would not have been possible without the encouragement, dedication, and expertise of many individuals and organizations.

First and foremost, we wish to thank our families for their unwavering love and support throughout the course of this endeavor. Their patience, understanding, and encouragement allowed us to navigate the challenges of writing and research, and their belief in the importance of this work kept us motivated even in the most difficult moments.

We would also like to thank our colleagues, collaborators, and mentors for their invaluable guidance and expertise. Their feedback, critiques, and suggestions throughout the writing process helped shape this book and ensured its accuracy and relevance. In particular, we would like to acknowledge the contributions of those who have provided expertise in the fields of postbiotic research, safety assessments, and therapeutic applications, which have significantly enriched the content of this book.

Our heartfelt thanks also go to Nova Science Publishers for their support and for providing the platform that enabled this project to come to fruition. Their professional expertise and encouragement have been essential to the completion of this work.

Lastly, we thank the readers, researchers, and students who will engage with this book. Your interest and dedication to advancing knowledge in medical bacteriology will continue to drive innovation in the field of postbiotics, ultimately improving human health and well-being.

We dedicate this book to the future of science and the individuals who will carry the torch forward, as they build upon the knowledge presented here to make even greater contributions to the field.

Preface

The human microbiome is a complex and dynamic ecosystem that plays a crucial role in our overall health and well-being. Over the past few decades, the growing body of research on probiotics, prebiotics, synbiotics, and postbiotics has revealed the profound impact that microorganisms have on various physiological processes, from digestion to immune function, and even mental health. The expanding field of medical bacteriology has opened up exciting possibilities for using these microbial products in therapeutic and preventive medicine.

"*Postbiotics in Medical Bacteriology*" aims to provide an in-depth exploration of the latest advancements in the understanding and application of postbiotics, which are non-viable microbial products and byproducts that have biological activity. These products, which include metabolic compounds like short-chain fatty acids (SCFAs), enzymes, peptides, and polysaccharides, hold significant potential for improving human health and managing diseases, without the risks associated with live probiotics.

The chapters of this book are designed to offer a comprehensive overview of the essential concepts related to postbiotics, beginning with the foundational understanding of probiotics, prebiotics, and synbiotics. We provide an in-depth look at the mechanisms of action of postbiotics, their safety assessments, preparation techniques, and their potential bio-utilization in the treatment of various medical conditions. By integrating the latest scientific research and providing practical insights, this work is intended to bridge the gap between basic microbiological studies and clinical applications.

We have drawn upon a wide range of studies and practical examples from across the world to highlight the relevance of postbiotics in medical bacteriology. This book will be particularly valuable to researchers, clinicians, and students in microbiology, immunology, pharmacology, and nutrition, who are interested in exploring how postbiotics can be harnessed for therapeutic purposes.

As we move toward an era where personalized medicine and microbiome-based therapies will be integral to healthcare, the importance of postbiotics in the development of new treatments and functional foods cannot be overstated. The promise of these microbial-derived compounds is vast, and we hope this book serves as a stepping stone for further research, deeper understanding, and practical application in improving human health.

We extend our sincere gratitude to all those who have contributed to the advancement of this field, and to the many individuals whose pioneering work continues to inspire us all.

Dr. Mahdi Asghari Ozma
asghariozma@gmail.com

Dr. Amin Abbasi
aminabasi.teh.ac.ir@gmail.com

Dr. Hossein Samadi Kafil
h.s.kafil@gmail.com

Chapter 1

The Probiotic Concept

Abstract

This chapter provides an overview of probiotics, highlighting their historical evolution, classifications, and significant health benefits. Probiotics are live microorganisms that confer health benefits when administered in adequate amounts. The chapter examines the origin of the term, its connection with ancient fermented foods, and the scientific advancements that have enabled modern understanding of probiotics. Special attention is given to well-researched strains, such as Lactobacillus and Bifidobacterium, and their role in gastrointestinal health, immune modulation, and overall well-being. Additionally, the mechanisms of action, including gut microbiota modulation and immune system regulation, are explored. The chapter concludes with a discussion of the potential therapeutic applications of probiotics in preventing and managing various diseases, including gastrointestinal, metabolic, and immune disorders.

Overview and History

Probiotics are viable microorganisms that, when administered in enough amounts, provide a health benefit to the host. It highlights the significance of these microorganisms' capability and quantity in achieving the intended health outcomes. Probiotics are primarily composed of bacteria, although some yeasts are also recognized as probiotics [1]. The term "probiotics" is derived from the Greek words "pro," meaning "for," and "bios," meaning "life." This etymology suggests that probiotics promote life, whereas "antibiotics" refers to "against life." Probiotics are commonly used in the form of fermented foods, which have been essential elements of human diets across various cultures for millennia. Yogurt, often included in many diets, is a rich source of probiotics, especially strains like *Lactobacillus bulgaricus* and *Streptococcus thermophilus*. Examples include kefir, a fermented dairy beverage with a diverse microbial composition, and kimchi, a traditional Korean dish composed of fermented vegetables celebrated for its probiotic benefits. Scientific advancements have significantly improved our comprehension of probiotics [2]. Researchers have found certain strains of bacteria and yeasts that provide distinct health benefits. An example is *Lactobacillus rhamnosus* GG, which has substantial evidence of its ability to prevent and treat gastrointestinal disorders. *Bifidobacterium lactis* is acknowledged for its capacity to enhance immune function. The mechanisms via which probiotics confer their beneficial effects are diverse and complex. Probiotics may modulate the gut microbiota, the community of microorganisms residing in the gastrointestinal tract [3].

Probiotics facilitate the growth of beneficial bacteria while inhibiting the proliferation of harmful bacteria, so maintaining a balanced gut microbiome is essential for overall health. In addition, probiotics increase the function of the intestinal barrier. They increase the production of mucins, glycoproteins that form a protective mucous layer on the intestinal lining. Additionally, they promote the synthesis of tight junction proteins that are essential for maintaining the integrity of the intestinal barrier [4]. This barrier prevents the transfer of harmful pathogens and toxins from the digestive system to the bloodstream. Probiotics also play a significant role in regulating the immune system. They interact with the gut-associated lymphoid tissue (GALT) and influence both innate and adaptive immune responses. Probiotics may enhance the production of anti-inflammatory cytokines while reducing the secretion of pro-inflammatory cytokines, helping to balance the immune system and reduce inflammation [5]. They also have a nutritional buoyancy in fermentation and production of short-chain fatty acids including butyrate, acetate, and propionate. Specific metabolites are synthesized by probiotic bacteria in the fermentation of dietary fibers. SCFAs provide various health benefits and are, among other things, the energy source of colonocytes and are involved in inflammatory and other reactions [6]. There is a lot of criticism and interest in probiotics due to their potential therapeutic applications. Many human studies have shown that various diseases can be prevented or treated using probiotics, most of which are digestive disorders, metabolic diseases, immune disorders, and mental health disorders. A growing number of studies show the benefits of probiotics in improving health and reducing the risk of disease. Probiotics are defined as significant fractions of microorganisms that, when introduced in effective amounts, have positive effects on the host. The use of probiotics in traditional cultures, along with the consumption of fermented foods since ancient times, points to the potential therapeutic role of these agents, alongside modern scientific progress in identifying specific strains and understanding their mechanisms.

Further research on probiotics reveals their potential to create new medicines and enhance human well-being [7].

The origins of probiotics can be linked back, to societies that predated the term "probiotics." Historical findings indicate that fermented foods were being eaten back as 6000 BCE by early settlers in regions like the Fertile Crescent, including parts of present-day Egypt and the Middle East where fermented dairy products were popularly consumed by the populace there long ago. These early civilizations realized that fermentation not only helped with food preservation but also enhanced flavors and provided health benefits to those who consumed them regularly. Throughout history, fermented foods have been a staple, in the diets of cultures worldwide [8]. Throughout history, nutritional habits in China and India have differed significantly. Fermented vegetables are a staple in Chinese cuisine, while yogurt and buttermilk are commonly consumed in India for their perceived health benefits. Hippocrates, the renowned Greek physician often regarded as the father of medicine, recognized the therapeutic properties of fermented milk for treating gastrointestinal disorders. Similarly, in ancient Rome, fermented dairy products were believed to aid digestion and promote overall well-being [9]. The organized investigation of probiotics started in the 1900s thanks to the work of Elie Metchnikoff. A scientist and Nobel Prize winner who conducted research at the Pasteur Institute, in Paris. Metchnikoff was intrigued by the long lifespan of farmers who regularly consumed fermented milk products. In 1907, he proposed that consuming fermented foods with lactic acid bacteria could improve health and extend life by reducing harmful bacteria in the gut. This discovery laid the foundation for modern research on probiotics. Other experts, such as Henry Tissier, continued to explore the beneficial effects of bacteria in fermented milk during the 1920s and 1930s. This French doctor discovered a special type of bacteria that colonized the digestive tract of infants and named it *Bifidobacterium*. He observed that these organisms are very abundant in the digestive system of healthy babies and suggested their use in the treatment of children's diarrhea [10]. Advanced methods in microbiology facilitated the isolation and typing of a large number of lactic acid bacteria (LAB) strains, including representatives of the genus *Lactobacillus*. However, these observations provided the basis for a deeper understanding of friendly bacteria in the human gastrointestinal tract and their possible therapeutic application. The study of probiotics effectively began after World War II, around the same time that antibiotics revolutionized the treatment of bacterial infections, revealing the side effects of disrupting gut flora [11]. In response, probiotics were used to restore the balance of gut flora. In the 1950s and 1960s, a Japanese scientist named Minoru Shirota developed a fermented milk drink called Yakult. This drink is made from a special strain of bacteria known as Lactobacillus casei Shirota. Shirota's contribution was crucial because his initiatives and efforts helped establish the production process and use of probiotic products. Yakult is considered one of the first probiotics to be commercially marketed. Probiotic research expanded significantly in the latter half of the 20th century and the early years of the 21st century, with researchers analyzing the complex two-way interactions between probiotics and the gut microbiota [12].

Recent knowledge in molecular biology and genetics has provided more information about how some probiotic bacteria work. Clinical evidence shows the effectiveness of probiotics in health conditions ranging from digestive disorders to immune system modulation and even mental health problems. Therefore, the increasing volume of data supports the development of probiotic supplements and functional foods that have made probiotics widely available to consumers [13]. Commercial success has paved the way for increased monitoring and the development of regulatory frameworks that ensure the safety and efficacy of probiotic products. Agencies such as the Food and Agriculture Organization (FAO) and the World Health Organization (WHO) provide guidance on the value and classification of probiotics. As a result, the global market for probiotics has grown significantly, spanning dietary supplements as well as probiotic-enriched foods and beverages. Rising consumer awareness about gut health and the importance of probiotics in maintaining overall health has further fueled this market [14].

Probiotics are also a very important area of research and development. Scientists are now focusing on studying new probiotic strains, understanding their mechanisms of action, and evaluating their possible applications in different conditions. Personalized probiotics, made for a specific microbiome profile, may represent a new frontier in this field of study. As medical science advances, the role of probiotics in both preventive health care and therapeutics should be tailored to provide specific interventional approaches to an unprecedented breadth of health and disease in humans. From ancient fermented foods to today's therapeutic probiotics, this journey reveals the unwavering role that good microbes play in health and wellness [15].

Types and Classification

Probiotics include various microorganisms, mainly bacteria and some yeasts, that have certain health benefits when consumed in sufficient amounts. Probiotics that are often studied and used belong to the genera *Lactobacillus* and *Bifidobacterium*. These bacteria produce lactic acid and create an acidic environment that prevents the proliferation of pathogenic microorganisms in the digestive tract [16]. *Lactobacillus* is a prominent genus of probiotics. Species such as *L. rhamnosus*, *Lactobacillus acidophilus*, and *L. casei* are distinguished by their ability to withstand the acidic conditions of the stomach and colonize the intestines. *L.rhamnosus* GG has been extensively studied for its efficacy in the prevention and treatment of gastrointestinal infections and diarrhea, particularly in pediatric populations [17]. *L. acidophilus* is known for its role in the degradation of lactose and its ability to reduce the symptoms of lactose intolerance. *Bifidobacterium* is an essential genus in the category of probiotics. Bifidobacterium longum, *Bifidobacterium bifidum*, and *B. lactis* are notable species known for their beneficial health benefits. *Bifidobacterium longum* helps balance the gut microbiota and is associated with improved digestion and immune function. *B. bifidum* is often found in the digestive tract of infants, which significantly aids in the digestion of complex carbohydrates and the synthesis of essential vitamins. *B. lactis* is associated with increased immune response and improved gut health [18] (Table 1).

Saccharomyces boulardii is one of the few yeast probiotics that set it apart from all bacterial probiotics. It is very effective in the prevention and treatment of various diarrheal diseases, such as antibiotic-associated diarrhea and traveler's diarrhea. Unlike bacterial probiotics, *S. boulardii* is resistant to antibiotics; thus, it is a good adjuvant to probiotic therapy, particularly for patients who are on antibiotic treatment [19]. Other important probiotic microorganisms are *S. thermophilus* and *Enterococcus faecium*. *S. thermophilus* is commonly used in yogurt and cheese production, enhancing the fermentation process and the product's probiotic properties. Although it is not considered a classic probiotic, *E. faecium* has gained some attention as an effective candidate for intestinal health, as well as prevention against gastrointestinal infections [20].

Table 1. Comprehensive classification of probiotics: genera, species, mechanisms, and applications

Genus	Species	Key Characteristics	Health Benefits	Mechanism of Action	Common Applications
Lactobacillus	*L. rhamnosus GG, L. acidophilus, L. casei*	Acid-resistant colonizes the intestines effectively	Enhances immune response, reduces diarrhea, aids lactose digestion	Modulates gut microbiota, promotes mucin production, strengthens gut barrier	Yogurt, kefir, dietary supplements
Bifidobacterium	*B. lactis, B. bifidum, B. longum*	Ferment dietary fibers synthesize essential vitamins	Balances gut flora, prevents constipation, boosts immune function	Produces SCFAs, supports beneficial microbial growth	Infant formulas, fermented dairy products
Saccharomyces	*S. boulardii*	Yeast-based probiotic, resistant to antibiotics	Prevents antibiotic-associated diarrhea, treats traveler's diarrhea	Competitive exclusion of pathogens supports the epithelial barrier	Probiotic supplements
Bacillus	*B. coagulans, B. subtilis*	Spore-forming bacteria survive harsh conditions	Supports digestion, modulates the immune system, reduces symptoms of IBS	Produces antimicrobial peptides, enhances gut health	Functional foods, probiotic beverages
Escherichia coli	*E. coli Nissle* 1917	Non-pathogenic strain, immunomodulatory properties	Treats ulcerative colitis, and reduces symptoms of irritable bowel syndrome	Competes with pathogens, enhances intestinal barrier function	Therapeutic formulations for IBD

Other emerging probiotics include various types of *Escherichia coli*, among which the highly regarded *E. coli* Nissle 1917 is used to treat inflammatory bowel diseases (IBD) such as ulcerative colitis. Spore-forming bacteria, such as *Bacillus coagulans* and *Bacillus subtilis*, are resistant to the harsh gastrointestinal environment, and their use has been explored for potential probiotic benefits [21].

The efficacy of probiotics is markedly strain-specific, indicating that not all strains within a genus have identical health advantages. This specialization requires meticulous selection and identification of strains for particular health outcomes. Progress in genetics and molecular biology is enabling the precise identification of probiotic strains, thereby facilitating the development of more effective probiotic treatments. Probiotic products are available in various formats, including nutritional supplements, functional foods, and beverages. While fermented foods like yogurt, kefir, sauerkraut, kimchi, and miso are traditional sources of probiotics, modern supplements often provide concentrated doses of specific strains [22]. The worldwide probiotic industry is expanding as research reveals further advantages and uses of these advantageous bacteria. In general, probiotics include various bacteria and yeasts that provide several health advantages. The most researched and used probiotics are from the genera *Lactobacillus* and *Bifidobacterium*, with significant input from *S. boulardii*, *S. thermophilus*, *E. faecium*, and developing strains of *E. coli* and *Bacillus* species. The specificity of probiotic effects underscores the importance of selecting suitable strains to achieve the desired health outcomes, while ongoing research continues to explore the full potential of these beneficial microbes in improving human health [23].

Novel Probiotic Strains

Recent developments in microbiome studies have come up with a very large number of new probiotic strains. These could provide health advantages not currently represented by classic strains like Lactobacillus and *Bifidobacterium*. These new probiotics are developed in various environments, exhibiting a wide range of characteristics that enhance digestive health, metabolic function, and even mental well-being. Therefore, it is essential to study these new varieties in depth to understand how they could facilitate future medical applications [24]. Until today, *Akkermansia muciniphila*, an intestinal mucin-degrading bacterium, was mostly present in the human gut. Therein, it can be presented as one of the most interesting new probiotic strains. Besides, *A. muciniphila* has also been involved in playing a significant role regarding the integrity of the gut mucosal barrier, something important for the prevention of pathogenic invasion for gut health [25]. Indeed, various studies have shown that *A. muciniphila* is inversely correlated with the prevalence of obesity, type 2 diabetes, and metabolic syndrome. *A. muciniphila* degrades mucin to produce beneficial compounds that regulate immune responses and enhance the function of the intestinal barrier. Potential medical applications of this strain include weight management, improvement of metabolic health, and possibly the mitigation of inflammatory diseases [26].

Table 2. Emerging probiotic strains and their novel applications

Strain	Unique Features	Targeted Health Benefits	Potential Applications
Akkermansia muciniphila	Mucin-degrading enhances gut barrier integrity	Reduces obesity, type 2 diabetes, and metabolic syndrome risks	Functional foods, personalized probiotic supplements
Faecalibacterium prausnitzii	Butyrate producer, anti-inflammatory properties	Prevents IBD, supports gut homeostasis	Treatments for Crohn's disease, ulcerative colitis
Clostridium butyricum	Anaerobic, produces SCFAs	Alleviates irritable bowel syndrome, antibiotic-associated diarrhea	Probiotic drugs for gastrointestinal health
Roseobacter spp.	Marine-derived, antimicrobial compounds	Combats inflammation, supports skin health	Novel antimicrobial therapies, skincare formulations

Also, *Faecalibacterium prausnitzii* is quite a good candidate to enter the probiotic rank. In the human gut, *F. prausnitzii* belongs to the most frequent butyrate-producing bacteria, being highly relevant in maintaining the gut's homeostasis. Butyrate is a short-chain fatty acid produced through the fermentation of dietary fibers. It serves as an energy source for colonocytes and has anti-inflammatory properties. Low levels of the bacterium *Faecalibacterium prausnitzii* have been associated with inflammatory bowel diseases (IBD), such as Crohn's disease and ulcerative colitis [27]. In addition, the genus *Clostridium* represents a new direction in the search for novel probiotic species. *Clostridium* butyricum is an anaerobic, butyrate-producing microorganism whose health benefits have been extensively studied. It has shown promise as a treatment for gastrointestinal issues, particularly irritable bowel syndrome (IBS) and antibiotic-associated diarrhea. Given its ability to produce butyrate and regulate the immune system, *C. butyricum* stands out as a strong contender in the development of probiotic therapies aimed at improving gut health and mitigating inflammation [28] (Table 2).

Other studies have also identified the possibility of certain strains of Escherichia coli being used as probiotics. One particular strain is the *E. coli* Nissle 1917, which has been more commonly referred to as EcN and has already been utilized medicinally for the past hundred years. EcN helps treat Gastrointestinal disorders such as ulcerative colitis and IBS because of its ability to competitively exclude pathogenic bacteria, modulate the immune response, and preserve gut barrier function. Even though *E. coli* is generally considered a disease-related bacterium, and its non-pathogenic strains, like EcN, have quite a few advantages to human health [29]. The *Bacillus* genus, which is well-known for its ability to create spores, involves many newly discovered probiotic species that have garnered much interest lately. Some of the most researched bacteria include *B. coagulans* and *B. subtilis*. Given that such strains can resist extreme environmental conditions, such as high temperatures and acidic media, they are well-suited for inclusion in a wide range of food products and dietary supplements. In the treatment of disorders like IBS, *B. coagulans* has proven effective, while *B. subtilis* has also shown potential in enhancing immune function and promoting gut health [30].

There are marine environments that have been identified as rich sources of new probiotic strains. Some of the specific characteristics of marine bacteria, such as Roseobacter and Alteromonas, have already been useful in human health. The same strains with the synthesis of bioactive compounds with antimicrobial and anti-inflammatory properties make these strains a good candidate for the development of a new probiotic drug. Besides affecting the healthy function of the stomach, some new probiotics influence mental health through their action on the gut-brain axis [31]. For example, symptoms of anxiety and depression can be alleviated by certain bacterial strains, such as *Bifidobacterium longum* and *Lactobacillus helveticus*. These probiotics are also considered supplementary treatments for mood disorders, as they may modulate neurotransmitters and reduce overall inflammation in the body. Additionally, a new generation of probiotics is currently under investigation for their potential effects on skin health. Presently, an experiment is in place based on knowing whether probiotic strains like *L. rhamnosus* and *S. thermophilus* possess the ability or capability to improve skin barrier function, reduce inflammation, and cure skin diseases such as eczema and acne. Further research is continuously being made to devise topical therapies as well as oral supplements employing these strains to improve the general health of skin from the inside out [32].

Table 3. Comprehensive overview of prebiotic types, sources, and benefits

Prebiotic Type	Natural Sources	Health Benefits	Role in Gut Health	Biological Effects
Fructooligosaccharides (FOS)	Garlic, onions, bananas, chicory root, asparagus	Promotes growth of beneficial gut bacteria, improves mineral absorption	Enhances mucosal health, supports microbiota balance	Increases Bifidobacteria and Lactobacilli, reduces harmful pathogens
Galactooligosaccharides (GOS)	Human milk, cow's milk derivatives	Supports infant gut microbiota, reduces IBS symptoms	Encourages growth of Bifidobacterium, enhances immune response	Produces SCFAs, reduces gut inflammation
Inulin	Leeks, garlic, bananas, chicory root, dandelion	Improves calcium absorption, regulates blood sugar, supports weight management	Stimulates SCFA production and strengthens gut barrier integrity	Enhances colonocyte energy, reduces pro-inflammatory cytokines
Resistant Starch	Green bananas, cooked and cooled potatoes, legumes	Improves insulin sensitivity, promotes satiety, reduces colon cancer risk	Produces SCFAs like butyrate, lowers gut inflammation	Modulates lipid metabolism, protects against oxidative stress
Xylooligosaccharides (XOS)	Bamboo, corn cobs, birch wood	Boosts immune function and reduces colon cancer risk	Selectively stimulates beneficial bacteria	Produces antimicrobial compounds, reduces systemic inflammation

On the contrary, despite several putative benefits attributed to new probiotic strains, it is emergently necessary to elaborate on the safety and efficacy in detail. Clinical trials and reviews of regulatory assessment studies will be required to ensure that such new probiotics are safe for consumption and are effective in providing the expected health outcomes. The progress in genomic and metagenomic technologies helps to describe those strains precisely, which will make the development of specialized probiotic medicines easier [33]. One of the biggest achievements so far in microbiome research has been the discovery and testing of new probiotic strains. *A. muciniphila, F. prausnitzii, Clostridium butyricum, E. coli* Nissle 1917, and various species of *Bacillus* all have the potential to improve intestinal health, metabolic function, and overall health (Table 3). The potential of these microbes is immense. Further research and development of probiotics could expand the range of beneficial bacterial therapies, offering new perspectives on enhancing human health through their microbial influence [34].

Chapter 2

The Prebiotic Concept

Abstract

This chapter delves into prebiotics, focusing on their role as non-digestible dietary components that selectively stimulate beneficial gut bacteria. The chapter defines prebiotics and their mechanisms of action, emphasizing how they contribute to improving gut health and overall well-being. Key types of prebiotics, such as fructooligosaccharides (FOS), galactooligosaccharides (GOS), inulin, and resistant starch, are discussed in detail along with their natural sources, health benefits, and physiological effects. Emerging prebiotics, including human milk oligosaccharides (HMOs) and xylooligosaccharides (XOS), are introduced as novel compounds that show promise for improving gut microbiota composition, supporting immune function, and mitigating metabolic diseases. The chapter concludes by highlighting the importance of prebiotics in modern nutrition and their potential therapeutic applications.

Introduction

Prebiotics are undigested dietary carbohydrates that beneficially affect the host by selectively stimulating the growth and/or activity of one or a limited number of colonic bacteria which leads to the improvement of host health. Unlike probiotics, which are living bacteria, prebiotics are complex carbohydrates or dietary fibers that the human digestive enzyme is unable to digest. Instead, they function as a nutrient source for beneficial bacteria harbored in the gut, thus stimulating their proliferation and activity [35]. In 1995, Glenn Gibson and Marcel Roberfroid were the first scientists to propose the concept of prebiotics. Prebiotics are defined as non-digestible dietary components that positively influence the host by selectively promoting the growth and/or activity of certain bacteria in the colon. This concept has been refined through subsequent research, expanding it to encompass a broader range of dietary fibers and oligosaccharides that may offer health benefits [36].

Types of Prebiotics

The majority of prebiotics are made up of oligosaccharides, which include fructooligosaccharides (FOS), galactooligosaccharides (GOS), inulin, and resistant starch. Each classification has a unique set of qualities and advantageous aspects. Composed of fructose molecules that are organized in SCFAs, FOS is a kind of sugar. These compounds may be found in their natural state in a wide range of plants, including onions, garlic, bananas, leeks, chicory root, and asparagus, among others. FOS has the potential to stimulate the growth of beneficial bacteria inside the gastrointestinal system, including Bifidobacteria and Lactobacilli, among other beneficial bacteria [37]. These beneficial microorganisms play a crucial role in maintaining the health of the digestive system by combating pathogenic bacteria and enhancing the protective function of the intestinal barrier. This is an essential factor in the preservation of digestive system health. Consistent consumption of FOS has been associated with improved gastrointestinal health, an improvement in the absorption of minerals namely calcium and magnesium, and the potential for the immune system to be strengthened. By increasing the amount of feces that are produced and the frequency with which they are produced, they may also help alleviate the symptoms of constipation [38].

Galactooligosaccharides, often known as GOS, are made up of short sequences of galactose molecules individually. It is essential for the development of the gut flora in infants that these chemicals be present in human milk, as they are naturally found in it. GOS can be produced from the lactose in cow's milk using enzymatic reactions. About the gastrointestinal system, GOS principally stimulates the growth of the beneficial bacteria Bifidobacteria. This may positively influence health in the gastrointestinal tract and help alleviate symptoms of gastrointestinal disorders, such as IBS. For instance, this treatment can reduce IBS symptoms. It has been concluded that GOS is a unique compound in gut organs and may enhance the immune system, potentially reducing susceptibility to infections and allergic reactions. The consumption of GOS during infancy may promote the development of a healthy gut microbiota and immune system, thereby potentially conveying beneficial outcomes similar to those associated with human milk oligosaccharides (HMOs) later in adult life [39].

Inulin is a type of polysaccharide made up of extended fructose molecules. It naturally occurs in chicory root, garlic, leeks, onions, dandelion root, and various types of vegetables, such as bananas and asparagus. Inulin is considered a prebiotic because of its ability to stimulate the growth of beneficial intestinal microbes. Inulin especially stimulates the growth of bifidobacteria. SCFAs are produced in the colon due to the fermentation process [40]. The primary component of the acids produced through this process is butyrate. The short-chain fatty acids (SCFAs) produced, in addition to their anti-inflammatory properties, serve as energy sources for the cells in the colon. Some of the associated beneficial effects of inulin include improved gastrointestinal regularity, enhanced calcium absorption, and potential weight management, among others. Additionally, inulin helps regulate blood sugar levels by slowing the digestion and absorption of carbohydrates into the bloodstream, where it plays a role in blood sugar management [41].

Resistant starch refers to starch that resists digestion within the small intestine and gets fermented in the large intestine. Some of its food sources are green bananas, cooked and cooled potatoes, lentils, and whole grains. Because it can trigger the proliferation of probiotic bacteria in the gut, resistant starch works as a prebiotic. The end products of this fermentation are short-chain fatty acids (SCFAs), which include butyrate, acetate, and propionate. These SCFAs have anti-inflammatory effects throughout the body and play a key role in maintaining gut health. Resistant starch has also been linked to improved insulin sensitivity, increased satiety, and a reduced risk of colon cancer. Additionally, two other potential benefits of this substance include regulating bowel movements and providing a significant boost to digestive system health [42].

Other Emerging Prebiotics

HMOs are complex carbohydrates found in human breast milk. They have a crucial role in shaping the gut microbiota of newborns, promoting the growth of beneficial bacteria such as *Bifidobacteria*. Despite the rarity of HMOs in adult diets, there is increasing interest in investigating their potential benefits in baby nutrition and maybe in adult health. Xylooligosaccharides (XOS) are oligosaccharides consisting of xylose monomers derived from plant sources, including bamboo, maize cobs, and birch wood. These chemicals may especially promote the proliferation of *Bifidobacteria* and *Lactobacilli*, hence benefiting gastrointestinal health [43]. Research has shown that XOS may enhance immunological function, increase mineral absorption, and perhaps reduce the risk of colon cancer development. Arabinoxylans are complex carbohydrates found in cereal grains, including wheat, rye, and barley [44]. They have prebiotic properties and may promote the growth of beneficial bacteria in the gastrointestinal system. Nowadays, studies on arabinoxylans investigate their role in improving gastrointestinal health, immune response, and metabolic health. Isomaltooligosaccharides (IMOs) are naturally occurring short chains of glucose molecules found in food items such as honey and fermented products. They possess prebiotic properties as they support the growth of beneficial microorganisms and improve gastrointestinal health. IMO is a low-calorie sweetener that has been associated with enhanced digestive health and the management of blood sugar levels [45] (Table 4).

Table 4. Key factors influencing probiotic efficacy

Factor	Description	Examples	Impact on Probiotic Performance
Strain Specificity	Different strains have unique effects	L. rhamnosus GG vs. *B. lactis*	Determines targeted health benefits
Dosage	Adequate CFU required for efficacy	Minimum of 10^6–10^9 CFU per dose	Low doses may not yield significant effects
Viability	Survival through the digestive tract	Enteric-coated capsules, spore-forming strains	Ensures delivery to the gut intact
Storage Conditions	Stability of live organisms	Refrigeration, freeze-drying	Poor storage reduces viability
Combination with Prebiotics	Enhances probiotic survival and colonization	Synbiotics with inulin or FOS	Maximizes health benefits

Examples of Prebiotics

Prebiotics are natural compounds found in various foods and vegetables, particularly those abundant in specific fibers and oligosaccharides. Nutrient-rich vegetables include garlic, onions, leeks, asparagus, chicory root, and dandelion greens. Inulin and FOS, present in significant amounts in garlic, promote the proliferation of beneficial bacteria in the digestive system. Onions also contain inulin and FOS, which support gastrointestinal health and enhance immune system functionality [46]. The consumption of leeks is associated with a considerable quantity of inulin, which plays a role in the multiplication of beneficial bacteria in the stomach. Asparagus, which is a rich source of the nutrient inulin, bolsters the health of the digestive tract and encourages regular bowel movements. Chicory root is the most abundant known source of inulin. Inulin is commonly used in dietary supplements and as an alternative to coffee. Dandelion greens are also rich in inulin and other forms of dietary fiber, which are beneficial for digestive health. Additionally, the resistant starch and FOS found in fruits like bananas, especially when they are unripe, are highly useful [47]. Pectin is a kind of fiber that also serves as a prebiotic, and apples are a rich source of pectin. Blueberries and raspberries are also sources of prebiotic fibers. Additionally, included in the category of prebiotic foods are barley, oats, wheat bran, flaxseeds, and chia seeds. Both beta-glucan and arabinoxylan, which are present in high concentrations of barley, are known to exhibit prebiotic characteristics [48]. Beta-glucan, which is found in substantial quantities in oats, stimulates the growth of beneficial bacteria in the stomach and provides several health benefits. Wheat bran contains arabinoxylan oligosaccharides, which are beneficial to the health of the digestive system or gastrointestinal tract. Mucilage is a type of fiber that forms a gel and functions as a prebiotic. Flaxseeds are rich in mucilage, while chia seeds are a source of soluble fiber, which is known for its prebiotic properties [49].

Foods belonging to the category of legumes, such as chickpeas, lentils, beans, and soybeans, offer a large amount of resistant starch and soluble fiber. These types of nutrients support the growth of good bacteria in the gut area. The chickpeas contain a significant amount of resistant starch and soluble fiber, which is believed to be an important promoter of gut health and intestinal regularity. Lentils contain a significant amount of prebiotic fibers. Most beans, including black beans, kidney beans, and navy beans, contain resistant starch and oligosaccharides, and are therefore considered prebiotics [50]. Oligosaccharides are also present in significant amounts within the structure of soybeans. They are responsible for the growth of microbes, which are useful to life forms. When it comes to prebiotic fiber, which is beneficial to the health of the gastrointestinal system, almonds and pistachios are both abundant sources. Additionally, pistachios are rich in prebiotic fibers that encourage the development of beneficial bacteria in the stomach, whilst almonds include prebiotic fiber that contributes to the maintenance of a healthy digestive tract [51]. The roots and tubers of certain plants, such as sweet potatoes, yams, and cassava (yuca), contain resistant starch along with various types of fibers that act as prebiotics. In addition to being rich in resistant starch, sweet potatoes also contain several different kinds of dietary fibers that serve as prebiotics. Yams, which share similar characteristics with sweet potatoes, also contain substantial quantities of prebiotic fibers. Cassava, which is often referred to as yuca, contains resistant starch and fiber, both of which are beneficial to the healthy functioning of the digestive system. Further sources of prebiotics include seaweeds like wakame and nori, which contain prebiotic fibers. Other sources of prebiotics include seaweed. The high fiber content of whole grains, such as rye and brown rice, is another reason why these grains are beneficial to the digestion process [52].

To incorporate foods that are high in prebiotics into your diet, you can substitute chicory root coffee, include raw garlic and onions in salads and dressings, cook and cool potatoes to increase the amount of resistant starch they contain, consume green bananas or use green banana flour, and if you have trouble consuming enough prebiotic foods, you might want to consider taking inulin supplements. Numerous foods and vegetables, particularly those that are abundant in certain types of fiber and oligosaccharides, include prebiotics. Prebiotics are found in such meals and vegetables [53]. By incorporating foods rich in prebiotic fibers into your diet, such as garlic, onions, leeks, chicory root, as well as fruits, grains, legumes, and nuts, you can significantly improve your overall health. Including a wide variety of these foods in your diet may help promote the growth of beneficial bacteria in your gut, improve digestive health, enhance immune system function, and yield numerous other positive health benefits [54].

Chapter 3

The Synbiotic Concept

Abstract

Synbiotics are combinations of probiotics and prebiotics that work synergistically to enhance the health benefits of both components. This chapter examines the concept of synbiotics, detailing the interplay between probiotics, which colonize the gut and modulate immune responses, and prebiotics, which stimulate the growth of beneficial bacteria. The mechanisms by which synbiotics improve gastrointestinal health, enhance gut barrier function, and modulate immune system activity are discussed. The chapter also explores the application of synbiotics in human health, animal nutrition, agriculture, and the food industry. The potential of synbiotics in treating gastrointestinal disorders, such as IBS, as well as their metabolic benefits in improving glucose metabolism and reducing inflammation, is examined. Lastly, the chapter explores challenges related to personalized approaches to synbiotic therapy.

Introduction

Synbiotics are a special mixture of probiotics and prebiotics, which in the last decade, have become one of the most talked-about subjects in gut health and general well-being studies. Synbiotics are also a mixture of probiotics and prebiotics. The objective of this combinatorial approach is to maximize the benefits derived from both components, which in turn enhances health through their combination. Probiotics are living microorganisms that provide health benefits when administered in adequate amounts. Prebiotics, on the other hand, are undigested nutritious substances that enable the proliferation and activity of beneficial bacteria living in the intestines. Both types of probiotics and prebiotics have been subjected to a significant amount of study. The combination of the two latter substances into synbiotics, however, is a form of therapy that proves to be more effective compared to the others [55]. Prebiotics promote the selective growth and activity of probiotics, which is a key mechanism that differentiates synbiotics from other forms of probiotics. By establishing this relationship, prebiotics ensure that the probiotics have a greater chance of surviving the harsh conditions within the gut and proliferating there. These prebiotics serve as a specific food source, enhancing the colonization and metabolic activity of probiotics, and consequently, their health benefits [56] (Table 5).

Table 5. Applications of synbiotics in various fields

Field	Application	Benefits	Examples
Human Health	Treating IBS, supporting immunity	Reduces inflammation, improves gut microbiota	L. rhamnosus + inulin
Animal Nutrition	Enhancing livestock health	Improves digestion, boosts growth rates	Probiotic-feed supplements
Agriculture	Soil health improvement	Promotes beneficial microbes, suppresses pathogens	Synbiotic-based fertilizers
Food Industry	Functional food production	Enhances product shelf-life, gut health benefits	Yogurt with added synbiotics
Pharmaceuticals	Drug development for chronic diseases	Reduces inflammation, improves metabolic function	Synbiotic capsules for diabetes

Synbiotics have been reported to positively influence several health aspects, including promoting the healthy functioning of the digestive system. Scholars have mostly focused on one benefit: the enhancement of gut microbial composition. Synbiotics enhance the population of beneficial bacteria, including *Bifidobacteria* and *Lactobacilli*, so supporting the maintenance of a healthy gut microbiome. The preservation of this balance is considered crucial for colonic health, as it helps prevent gastrointestinal disorders such as diarrhea, IBS, and IBD. Moreover, synbiotics have been shown to significantly improve intestinal barrier function [57]. The gut barrier is a vital structure that protects against the entry of harmful pathogens and chemicals from the digestive tract into the bloodstream. Synbiotics strengthen this barrier to further help fight off infections, which contributes to a decline in inflammation and danger from systemic infections. Synbiotics also help to kill the risk of infection. A technique like this might dramatically benefit people with leaky gut syndrome condition where the barrier protecting the gut is destroyed. Another critical point to note is that synbiotics have been shown to modulate the immune system. GALT (Gut-associated lymphoid tissue) plays a crucial role in immunity. It has been observed that synbiotics enhance the function of GALT, thereby improving the body's immune responses (Table 6). This is particularly important in reducing the incidence of infections, allergies, and autoimmune diseases, as well as their severity [58].

Table 6. Comparison of probiotics, prebiotics, and synbiotics

Feature	Probiotics	Prebiotics	Synbiotics
Definition	Live microorganisms provide health benefits	Non-digestible fibers promote beneficial bacteria growth	Combination of probiotics and prebiotics for enhanced effects
Key Examples	*Lactobacillus, Bifidobacterium, Saccharomyces*	Inulin, FOS, GOS, resistant starch	*L. rhamnosus* + inulin, B. lactis + FOS
Primary Mechanism	Colonization of the gut, immune modulation	Feeding gut bacteria, SCFA production	Supports probiotic survival and activity
Benefits	Improved digestion, reduced inflammation	Enhanced microbiota balance, gut health	Combined benefits of probiotics and prebiotics
Applications	Fermented foods, dietary supplements	Fiber-rich diets, functional foods	Supplements for gastrointestinal and metabolic health

The potential metabolic benefits further complement the prebiotic and probiotic effects of synbiotics. Indeed, several studies have shown that synbiotics can positively modulate lipid metabolism, potentially reducing the risk of cardiovascular disease. Moreover, they have been associated with improved glucose metabolism and insulin sensitivity, both of which may benefit individuals who are already suffering from or are at risk of developing type 2 diabetes. Additionally, synbiotics have also shown promise in the field of mental health. The gut-brain axis is an important constituent in the regulation of mood and cognitive performance due to its bidirectional communication between the stomach and the brain. Synbiotics may thus have beneficial influences on symptoms related to anxiety, stress, and depression by acting positively on gut microbiota. Results obtained from several researches indicate that synbiotics can improve cognitive function and reduce the risk of neurodegenerative illnesses involved in Alzheimer's disease. On the subject of their uses, synbiotics have many usages other than in human health [59].

Recently, synbiotics have emerged as a prospective strategy in the agricultural field to enhance animal health and productivity. The use of synbiotics is expected to contribute to increasing growth rate, feed efficiency, and animal welfare in cattle. The likely reason is that synbiotics enhance the health of the gastrointestinal system and nutrient absorption in cattle. In other words, this could lead to significant economic advantages for rural communities in the agricultural sector. While synbiotics hold great potential, several challenges and factors must be considered. Nevertheless, synbiotics remain highly promising. The effectiveness of synbiotics may vary, as the probiotics and prebiotic strains used in the synbiotic combination may differ. This is relative to the individual variability in the gut for the composition of microbiota. Due to this, it may be that customized approaches are required to maximize the benefits imposed by synbiotics [60].

Chapter 4

Postbiotics and Paraprobiotics

Abstract

This chapter explores postbiotics and paraprobiotics, focusing on their role as non-viable bacterial products and inactivated microbial cells, respectively. Postbiotics, including metabolic byproducts such as peptides, enzymes, and short-chain fatty acids (SCFAs), are discussed for their biological activities and stability compared to live probiotics. Their immunomodulatory, anti-inflammatory, and pathogen-suppressing effects are highlighted, along with their potential advantages in treating vulnerable populations, such as immunocompromised individuals. Paraprobiotics, defined as inactivated probiotic cells, are also examined for their ability to interact with the immune system and provide health benefits without the risks associated with live bacteria. The chapter concludes with an exploration of psychobiotics, immunobiotics, and proteobiotics as subcategories of postbiotics with promising therapeutic potentials, particularly in mental health and immune modulation.

Postbiotics

Probiotics are the organisms that are responsible for the fermentation process, which ultimately leads to the formation of postbiotics, which are helpful compounds. Probiotics are live microorganisms, while postbiotics are metabolic byproducts or non-viable bacterial products that are created by probiotic microorganisms and exhibit biologically active features. Probiotics are a kind of bacterium that is considered to be beneficial to the body. Enzymes, peptides, teichoic acids, muropeptides formed from peptidoglycan, polysaccharides, cell surface proteins, and organic acids such as SCFAs all fall into this category. It also includes a broad range of muropeptides. The concept of postbiotics originated from the realization that the benefits offered by probiotics may be attributed not only to the live bacteria themselves but also to the substances they produce. This realization led to the development of postbiotics [61].

There are a variety of biological acts that postbiotics may perform, some of which include immunomodulatory effects, anti-inflammatory capabilities, pathogen suppression, and the maintenance of the integrity of the intestinal barrier. Another advantage of postbiotics over probiotics is that they are more stable than probiotics. This is one of the key advantages of postbiotics. Probiotics are generally more resilient to adverse environmental conditions, such as heat, pH variations, and exposure to oxygen, due to their inherent adaptive mechanisms. These mechanisms enable them to survive and maintain their viability under stressful conditions that would otherwise affect their metabolic activity and overall functionality [62]. As non-living entities, they are less susceptible to these conditions, making them less sensitive to environmental stressors. As a result of this, postbiotics are particularly desirable when they are included in a wide range of products, such as meals, beverages, and supplements. Additionally, the risk of infection or translocation that is connected with live microorganisms is not present with postbiotics. This is because postbiotics are not living organisms. The presence of this characteristic renders postbiotics more suitable for use in vulnerable populations, including immunocompromised individuals, infants, and the elderly [63].

Paraprobiotics

Paraprobiotics refer to inactivated microbial cells that, despite not being alive, can still provide health benefits to the host. These cells are also commonly referred to as non-viable probiotics or 'ghost probiotics.' The concept of paraprobiotics is based on the discovery that even non-viable bacteria can interact with the host's immune system and produce beneficial effects. This interaction is facilitated by various components within the bacterial cell, such as cell wall fragments, surface proteins, and nucleic acids, which are believed to play key roles in mediating these health benefits. Deoxyribonucleic acid (DNA), the proteins on the cell surface, and fragments of the cell wall are all examples of these components [64]. These components may potentially boost the immune system, enhance gut barrier function, and regulate the microbiota in the gut. The inactivation of probiotics, which is necessary for the production of paraprobiotics, can be achieved through various methods, including freeze-drying, heat treatment, and UV irradiation. These methods must be used to get the desired results. Although the benefits of paraprobiotics are similar to those of probiotics and postbiotics, they are distinguished by a higher degree of safety and stability than their counterparts [65].

Since paraprobiotics are non-living organisms, they reduce the likelihood of live bacteria becoming infected, overgrowing, or migrating to different locations. These characteristics make paraprobiotics particularly suitable for use in individuals with compromised immune systems, as well as in infants and the elderly. Additionally, compared to live probiotics, paraprobiotics are more stable, which facilitates their inclusion in a broader range of products. However, it is important to note that the health benefits of paraprobiotics are strain-specific, meaning not all strains retain their therapeutic properties after inactivation. Therefore, careful strain selection and validation are crucial to ensure their effectiveness and support overall health maintenance [66].

Psychobiotics

Psychobiotics is a compelling and rapidly evolving area of research that connects gastrointestinal health with psychological well-being. These microorganisms, mostly including certain strains of probiotics and their metabolites, have attracted interest for their capacity to affect the gut-brain axis and enhance mental health. The concept of psychobiotics was first introduced in 2013 and has since evolved as researchers continue to uncover the significant influence of gut microbes on the central nervous system [67]. This complex interaction highlights the importance of a healthy gut microbiota in maintaining cognitive and emotional well-being. The gut-brain axis functions as a crucial communication channel linking the gastrointestinal system to the brain via a network of neuronal, endocrine, and immunological systems [68]. The vagus nerve, one of the longest nerves in the body, plays a crucial role in transmitting information between the gastrointestinal tract and the brain. Additionally, intestinal microbiota produce neurotransmitters and neuroactive substances, such as serotonin, dopamine, GABA, and SCFAs, which directly influence brain function and emotional states. Over 90% of the body's serotonin, a key neurotransmitter involved in mood regulation, is synthesized in the gut, underscoring the vital importance of gut health for emotional well-being [69].

Psychobiotics influence their effects by altering gut microbiota composition, increasing the synthesis of neuroactive compounds, and diminishing inflammation. Chronic inflammation and heightened intestinal permeability, have been associated with several neuropsychiatric illnesses, including depression, anxiety, and autism spectrum disorders [70]. Psychobiotics enhance intestinal barrier integrity and reduce systemic inflammation, creating a healthier environment that supports optimal brain function. Additionally, these beneficial bacteria interact with immune cells and regulate cytokine production, thereby influencing mental health. The potential applications of psychobiotics in the treatment of mental health disorders are vast. Numerous clinical trials have shown their effectiveness in mitigating symptoms of despair and anxiety [71]. Strains such as *Lactobacillus helveticus* R0052 and *Bifidobacterium longum* R0175 have shown the ability to lower cortisol levels, a stress biomarker, and enhance mood in human studies. Lactobacillus rhamnosus JB-1 has been shown to increase GABA receptor expression in the brain, hence diminishing anxiety-like behaviors. Psychobiotics' capacity to affect these pathways underscores their potential as supplementary treatments for conventional psychotropic medicines [72].

Besides their influence on mood problems, psychobiotics may contribute to cognitive improvement. Studies indicate that certain strains may enhance memory and learning capabilities by regulating brain-derived neurotrophic factor (BDNF), a protein essential for synaptic plasticity and neurogenesis. Research has provided compelling data on the cognitive benefits of psychobiotics, and emerging human trials are beginning to support similar findings [73]. This opens new possibilities for addressing neurodegenerative disorders like Alzheimer's and Parkinson's, where inflammation and gut dysbiosis play key roles. Psychobiotics also have the potential to improve stress resilience. Chronic stress alters gut microbiota composition and facilitates the development of mood disorders. Psychobiotics may mitigate the detrimental effects of stress on the gut and brain by reinstating microbial diversity and fostering the proliferation of beneficial bacteria. Moreover, these microbes generate metabolites like as SCFAs, which possess anti-inflammatory characteristics and facilitate the synthesis of neuroprotective substances [74].

Diet and lifestyle significantly influence the gut microbiota, and integrating psychobiotics into everyday routines via functional foods or supplements provides a pragmatic method for enhancing mental health. Fermented foods including yogurt, kefir, sauerkraut, and kimchi inherently contain advantageous bacteria that function as psychobiotics. Targeted supplementation with certain strains may be more efficacious for those with significant gut dysbiosis or specific mental health issues [75]. The safety profile of psychobiotics is generally positive, as they originate from naturally occurring microbes in the human gastrointestinal tract. This makes them suitable for use across various demographics, including children, the elderly, and immunocompromised individuals. However, the strain-specific characteristics of psychobiotic effects require careful strain selection and clinical validation to ensure both effectiveness and safety. Not all probiotics are classified as psychobiotics, and their capacity to affect mental health is contingent upon criteria such as viability, dose, and metabolic activity [76].

Immunobiotics

Immunobiotics are a distinct subset of probiotics recognized for their capacity to influence the immune system. These advantageous bacteria affect both innate and adaptive immune responses, enhancing host defense against infections and improving the management of immunological-mediated diseases. The name "immunobiotics" underscores their dual function as probiotics with immunomodulatory characteristics, making them an essential asset in enhancing health and averting illnesses. The immune system is a complex network of cells, tissues, and chemicals that defends the body against infections while maintaining tolerance to harmless antigens, such as dietary proteins and commensal bacteria [77]. Immunobiotics interact with various components of the immune system, including GALT, the body's largest immune organ. They influence immune responses by engaging with immune cells, such as macrophages, dendritic cells, and T cells [78, 79].

Immunobiotics primarily exert their effects by regulating cytokine production. These bacteria can enhance the synthesis of anti-inflammatory cytokines, such as interleukin-10 (IL-10), while inhibiting pro-inflammatory cytokines, such as TNF-α. This immunoregulatory function helps maintain immunological homeostasis and prevents excessive inflammation, which is often associated with chronic conditions like IBD and rheumatoid arthritis. Immunobiotics play a significant role in strengthening the body's defense against infections [80]. Specific strains, including *L.plantarum*, *L.rhamnosus*, and *B.bifidum*, have shown the ability to enhance the gut barrier by elevating the synthesis of tight junction proteins and mucus. This improved barrier function inhibits the transfer of detrimental microorganisms and poisons into the circulation. Moreover, immunobiotics may stimulate PRRs, including TLRs, in immune cells, resulting in the synthesis of antimicrobial peptides and the mobilization of immune cells to areas of infection [81].

The advantages of immunobiotics beyond the gastrointestinal system. Research has shown their capacity to influence respiratory and systemic immune responses. Immunobiotics have shown the ability to mitigate the severity of respiratory infections by augmenting mucosal immunity in the respiratory system. This positions them as a promising alternative for the prevention and management of ailments such as the common cold, influenza, and severe respiratory infections. Immunobiotics are being investigated for their potential in controlling allergies and autoimmune disorders [82]. These probiotics may alleviate hypersensitivity reactions and autoimmune responses by enhancing regulatory T cell (Treg) activity and restoring immunological balance. Recent data indicates that some strains may alleviate symptoms of allergic rhinitis, asthma, and atopic dermatitis by regulating immune responses and enhancing gut health. The safety and efficiency of immunobiotics are contingent upon the individual strain used since their immunomodulatory characteristics are unique to each strain. Clinical experiments have emphasized the importance of selecting and identifying strains with demonstrated immunobiotic potential. Moreover, their use in functional foods, dietary supplements, and medications is becoming increasingly popular, offering a natural and preventative approach to supporting immunological health [83].

Proteobiotics

Proteobiotics represent a novel idea in microbiology and biotechnology, emphasizing the use of protein-based metabolites sourced from probiotics to provide health advantages. Bioactive proteins and peptides generated by the fermentation or metabolic activity of probiotic microbes are essential for enhancing human health by affecting several physiological systems. The word "proteobiotics" emphasizes their distinct role as protein-focused bioactives, setting them apart from the wider classifications of probiotics and postbiotics [84]. A key characteristic of proteobiotics is their antibacterial efficacy. Numerous proteobiotic substances, including bacteriocins and antimicrobial peptides, are excreted by probiotic bacteria to suppress the proliferation of rival pathogens. Bacteriocins produced by *Lactobacillus* and *Bifidobacterium* strains specifically target pathogenic bacteria by compromising their cell membranes, hence decreasing the likelihood of infections in the gastrointestinal tract and other mucosal surfaces. These natural antimicrobial compounds provide a viable alternative to conventional antibiotics, particularly in light of increasing antibiotic resistance [85].

Proteobiotics possess notable immunomodulatory characteristics. Specific peptides secreted by probiotics can interact with immune cells, including macrophages and dendritic cells, to modulate cytokine production. Some proteobiotic peptides promote the secretion of anti-inflammatory cytokines, while others enhance the immune response to combat infections. The dual functionality of proteobiotics makes them significant in the management of inflammatory diseases, such as IBD, and in boosting host immunity [86]. A vital component of proteobiotics is their contribution to gastrointestinal health and integrity. Proteins and peptides from probiotics support the integrity of the intestinal barrier by enhancing the synthesis of tight junction proteins, which inhibit the entry of hazardous chemicals and pathogens into the circulation. Moreover, some proteobiotics may bind to intestinal receptors, thereby regulating gut-brain communication and influencing neurological function. The connection between the gut-brain axis suggests potential applications of proteobiotics in the treatment of anxiety, depression, and other neuroinflammatory disorders [87].

Beyond their obvious health advantages, proteobiotics are becoming recognized for their impact on metabolic health. Probiotic-derived proteins and peptides have shown efficacy in enhancing insulin sensitivity, modulating lipid metabolism, and mitigating inflammation linked to metabolic diseases. Proteobiotics may affect signaling pathways linked to energy balance, presenting therapeutic promise for the management of obesity, diabetes, and other metabolic disorders. The creation and characterization of proteobiotics require advanced methods, such as proteomics and bioinformatics [88]. Identifying the precise protein molecules and understanding their modes of action are crucial for fully comprehending their therapeutic potential. Research efforts are focused on improving the fermentation process to optimize the production of proteobiotics and ensure their stability across various delivery forms, including functional foods, beverages, and supplements. Despite their potential applications, the development of proteobiotics faces challenges, such as strain-specific variability and ensuring their safety for consumption [86].

Chapter 5

The Classification of Functional Postbiotics

Abstract

This chapter provides a comprehensive classification of functional postbiotics, focusing on their diverse biological roles and therapeutic applications. Postbiotics, including supernatants from bacterial fermentation, antioxidant enzymatic components, and exopolysaccharides, are explored in terms of their bioactive properties. The chapter emphasizes the production and potential of short-chain fatty acids (SCFAs) in enhancing gut health, immune function, and metabolic regulation. Key bioactive molecules in postbiotics, such as bacteriocins and antimicrobial peptides, are discussed for their role in pathogen inhibition and immune system modulation. The chapter concludes by detailing the use of postbiotics in the management of gastrointestinal diseases, metabolic disorders, and immune-related conditions, underscoring their growing importance in functional food and therapeutic applications.

Supernatants Obtained from Cellular Fractions

Recent advancements in microbiome research have progressed beyond the examination of probiotics to investigate a wider array of bioactive substances, collectively known as postbiotic molecules. Supernatants derived from cellular fractions have garnered considerable interest owing to their varied and powerful biological effects. Supernatants are the liquid byproducts of bacterial fermentation, including a combination of beneficial chemicals generated by probiotic microbes. This study will provide a comprehensive analysis of the composition, modes of action, and prospective therapeutic uses of these supernatants, emphasizing their potential as a feasible technique for producing novel health solutions. Supernatants are intricate combinations obtained from the cellular components of probiotic bacteria [89]. Supernatants contain a wide array of bioactive compounds, including metabolites such as SCFAs, peptides, enzymes, polysaccharides, teichoic acids, and cell surface proteins. The specific composition of these supernatants can vary significantly depending on factors such as bacterial strain, growth conditions, and fermentation substrates. SCFAs, including acetate, propionate, and butyrate, are commonly found in these supernatants and have been associated with beneficial effects on gut health and metabolism. Additionally, supernatants often contain bacteriocins and antimicrobial peptides (AMPs) produced by bacteria, which play a key role in inhibiting infections. These properties underscore the potential of supernatants as valuable agents for promoting health and combating infections [90].

Various bioactive compounds are present in the supernatants exhibiting diverse modes of action. As one such example, SCFAs stimulate the production of tight junction proteins, thereby enhancing gut barrier integrity by reducing intestinal permeability. It acts to obstruct the passage of harmful bacteria and noxious chemicals from the intestines into the circulation to prevent such substances' movement. The more common gastrointestinal illnesses related to this condition are IBD and leaky gut syndrome. Due to anti-inflammatory action and the fact that they represent a source of energy for colonocytes, SCFAs represent essential players in the maintenance processes of the intestinal epithelium. It is also possible that peptides and enzymes are present in this liquid fraction, which may influence immune responses. Some peptides function as signaling molecules that interact with immune cells by promoting anti-inflammatory cytokines and suppressing the production of pro-inflammatory cytokines. This chemical immunomodulatory action helps maintain the balance of the immune system and may therefore be beneficial in conditions characterized by chronic inflammation of tissues, such as allergic and autoimmune diseases [91]. The presence of exopolysaccharides, more so polysaccharides, in the supernatants, is very crucial to ensure the attachment of the beneficial bacteria to the gut mucosa, thereby enhancing the capacity of the bacteria to establish and sustain a presence in the gut. The polysaccharides can serve as prebiotics, that is, they can stimulate the growth of beneficial bacteria in the gut microbiota. This, in turn, contributes to the development of a well-balanced and healthy microbial ecology. Teichoic acids and cell surface proteins can modulate the host's immune system, thus improving the ability of the host immune system to recognize and effectively respond against dangerous infections. Some interactions can enhance the activity of immune cells, which include macrophages, dendritic cells, and other immune cells, and thus enhance the body's defense mechanisms [92].

Supernatants formed from cellular fractions possess a variety of biological roles that indicate much promise for many different therapeutic applications. Among the areas that have garnered the most attention from researchers is their potential to successfully treat gastrointestinal illnesses. These supernatants may improve symptoms and lead to better patient outcomes in conditions like IBS, IBD, and diarrhea by restoring gut barrier integrity and modulating immune responses. One empirical study has documented the potential of supernatants derived from certain probiotic strains in reducing inflammation, aiding the regeneration of the mucosal lining, and restoring the balance of microbiota of the gut of those persons affected by such illnesses. Apart from the influence of supernatants on health in the gastrointestinal tract, it has also been suggested that they are capable of affecting metabolic processes [93]. More precisely, it has been suggested that SCFAs play a role in enhancing insulin sensitivity and, further, in lipid metabolism. These supernatants may be beneficial in managing metabolic disorders like obesity and type 2 diabetes due to their ability to influence the secretion of hormones involved in regulating appetite and glucose balance, such as Glucagon-like peptide 1 (GLP-1) and peptide YY (PYY). Animal studies, along with pilot human trials, have shown a reduction in body weight, improved glycemic control, and lower circulating lipid levels following supplementation with supernatants [94, 95].

Besides this, the supernatants being immunomodulatory also make them a very attractive candidate in the treatment of immune-related disorders. Their potential in enhancing anti-inflammatory cytokine production and inhibiting pro-inflammatory cytokine production may be helpful in the treatment of autoimmune diseases like rheumatoid arthritis and multiple sclerosis [96]. Besides that, supernatants contain an antimicrobial peptide, which naturally fights infection. This limits the use of conventional antibiotics, thereby reducing the risk of antibiotic resistance. Supernatants have also been shown to improve skin health. Formulations containing these supernatants have been developed as topical treatments for skin conditions such as acne, eczema, and psoriasis. Their anti-inflammatory and antibacterial properties help reduce skin irritation and inhibit the growth of harmful bacteria, promoting healthier skin [97].

The production of the supernatant would involve growing the probiotic bacteria under controlled conditions, after which the bacterial cells are removed from the liquid fraction. This can be modified to adapt to specific demands to enhance the functionality of the liquid fraction and the chemical nature of the bioactive substances. The quality and efficacy of the supernatants depend upon the selected bacterial strain, growth medium, time course of fermentation, and environmental factors such as temperature and pH. There is a high need for standardization of the supernatant to ensure the effectiveness of treatment consistently. It calls for the quantification of the essential bioactive compounds as well as the establishment of quality control methodologies to check the stability and activity of the reagents. Advanced analytical methodologies used to analyze supernatants include techniques such as high-performance liquid chromatography (HPLC), mass spectrometry, and nuclear magnetic resonance (NMR) spectroscopy. These methods enable the determination of the supernatants' composition and ensure that the results are consistent and not dependent on batch variations [98] (Table 7).

Table 7. Therapeutic applications of supernatants from cellular fractions

Condition	Mechanism of Action	Key Bioactive Compounds	Therapeutic Benefits	Example Applications
Gastrointestinal Disorders	Restores gut barrier integrity, modulates immune response	SCFAs (butyrate, acetate), peptides	Reduces IBS symptoms, enhances gut health	Treatment for IBD, IBS
Metabolic Syndrome	Enhances insulin sensitivity, regulates lipid metabolism	GLP-1, PYY, SCFAs	Improves glucose metabolism, reduces obesity risk	Metabolic disorder supplements
Immune-Related Diseases	Promotes anti-inflammatory cytokines	Teichoic acids, cell surface proteins	Decreases inflammation, improves autoimmune condition management	Treatment for rheumatoid arthritis
Skin Conditions	Antimicrobial, anti-inflammatory effects	Exopolysaccharides, enzymes	Reduces acne, eczema, and psoriasis	Topical creams for skin health
Infectious Diseases	Inhibits pathogenic growth, boosts host defense	Bacteriocins, antimicrobial peptides	Prevents infections, reduces antibiotic dependence	Antibiotic-alternative therapies

There are major safety and regulatory considerations associated with the use of supernatants obtained from cellular fractions. Since these supernatants arise from bacterial fermentation processes, it becomes very critical that they do not contain injurious contaminants, which include endotoxins, mycotoxins, and residual bacterial cells. Stringent purification with quality control processes will be highly important in assuring the safety of the product for human consumption. The research and refinement of the regulatory frameworks for postbiotics, including supernatants, is a continuous process. Postbiotics are relatively new, and a set of guidelines to be followed needs to be put in place to ensure their safety and efficacy. This is in comparison to the regulatory mechanisms that have been so well laid out for probiotics and prebiotics [99]. The U.S. Food and Drug Administration (FDA), in collaboration with the European Food Safety Authority (EFSA), is currently developing a set of criteria and guidelines for the evaluation and approval of postbiotic products. These guidelines are expected to address key issues related to safety, efficacy, labeling, and claims, thereby establishing a regulatory framework for the marketing of products derived from supernatant components [100].

Antioxidant Enzymatic Components

Antioxidant enzymatic components represent major improvements in the use of postbiotics within microbiome research and their therapeutic applications. The concept of postbiotics goes beyond the typical probiotics that are comprised of living microorganisms but include non-viable bacterial metabolites or metabolic byproducts that confer health benefits. The antioxidant enzymatic components are considered some of the most promising constituents of these postbiotic substances, given their ability to reduce oxidative stress. Oxidative stress refers to a condition in which there is an imbalance between the production of reactive oxygen species (ROS) and the body's antioxidant defenses. Antioxidant enzymes have henceforth emerged as one of the priority areas of research and development since such oxidative stress is linked with various chronic diseases: cardiovascular diseases, neurological disorders, diabetes, and even cancer [101].

ROS, are extremely reactive molecules. These include free radicals such as superoxide anion and hydroxyl radical, and non-radical species such as hydrogen peroxide. These chemicals are produced during normal cellular metabolism and are essential for cell signaling and maintaining homeostasis.

On the other hand, excess ROS can cause oxidative damage to cellular biomolecules such as DNA, proteins, and lipids, leading to impaired cellular functions that may contribute to the development of diseases. Antioxidant enzymes, including superoxide dismutase (SOD), catalase (CAT), and glutathione peroxidase (GPx), play a crucial role in neutralizing ROS and protecting cells from oxidative damage [102] (Table 8).

Table 8. Functions and sources of antioxidant enzymatic components in postbiotics

Enzyme	Source	Function	Health Benefits	Applications
Superoxide Dismutase (SOD)	Lactobacillus, Bifidobacterium strains	Neutralizes superoxide radicals	Reduces oxidative stress, prevents cellular damage	Cardiovascular health, neuroprotection
Catalase (CAT)	Fermentation by probiotics	Decomposes hydrogen peroxide into water and oxygen	Prevents chronic inflammation, enhances tissue repair	Supplements for oxidative stress management
Glutathione Peroxidase	Enzymatic extracts from probiotic cultures	Converts hydrogen peroxide into non-toxic substances	Protects DNA, proteins, and lipids from damage	Diabetes management, anti-aging therapies
Peroxidases	Postbiotic supernatants	Reduces ROS	Supports immune function, delays aging processes	Functional foods, pharmaceutical formulations

In this reaction, superoxide anion is transformed into oxygen and hydrogen peroxide through a catalyzing action utilizing an enzyme called SOD. This provides an important first line of defense against oxidative stress. Next, hydrogen peroxide is degraded into water and oxygen by the action of CAT, further reducing the concentration of ROS. Glutathione peroxidase, or GPx, represents a group of enzymes with glutathione as the substrate. The enzyme catalyzes the following reactions: the reduction of hydrogen peroxide to water and the reduction of organic hydroperoxides to their corresponding alcohols. Enzymatically, these reactions work together to maintain the cellular redox state and detoxify reactive oxygen species (ROS), thereby protecting against oxidative damage to cellular components. Lactic acid bacteria (LAB), which are probiotic microorganisms, generally produce various bioactive substances during fermentation, including antioxidant enzymes. These enzymatic components may be extracted from probiotic cultures and used as postbiotics. The production process involves the growth of the probiotic strains under optimal conditions to enhance the availability of the enzymes [103]. This is followed by the separation of bacterial cells from the culture medium and the subsequent isolation of enzymatic components from the supernatant. However, the exact composition of these components, as well as the yield, may vary depending on the strain of bacteria used, the growth conditions, and the fermentation substrates. Spectrophotometric assays, zymography, and mass spectrometry are some of the methods used to quantify and identify antioxidant enzymes in the supernatant following fermentation [104].

There are several different routes by which the antioxidant enzymatic components exhibit their effects. First, they immediately neutralize ROS, which prevents oxidative damage to the components of the cell. They protect DNA, proteins, and lipids from oxidative stress by transforming ROS into molecules with a lower level of reactivity. These enzymes, in the second place, are responsible for modulating redox signaling pathways, which are responsible for regulating a variety of cellular processes such as inflammation, apoptosis, and cell proliferation. The anti-inflammatory and cytoprotective actions of antioxidant enzymatic components may be attributed to their ability to influence the redox signaling pathway. Additionally, these enzymes can enhance the body's natural antioxidant defenses by promoting the synthesis of essential intracellular antioxidants like glutathione. This is achieved through the activation of transcription factors such as nuclear factor erythroid 2-related factor 2 (Nrf2), which regulate the production of these antioxidants. In summary, enzymatic antioxidant components can interact with gut microbiota, promoting balance in the gut's microbial ecology and boosting the overall antioxidant capacity of the gut environment [105]. Because of their potentially powerful antioxidant characteristics, enzymatic components produced from probiotics may be utilized in a wide range of therapeutic manners. It has been regarded as one of the major factors in the development of cardiovascular illnesses, such as atherosclerosis, hypertension, and heart failure, concerning the health of the cardiovascular system. Antioxidant enzymatic components, thus, might theoretically reduce the incidence of cardiovascular events by mitigating oxidative damage occurring in blood vessels and heart tissue. Various studies have determined these enzymes exert an endothelium-enhancing action, lipid peroxidation reduction, and inhibition of atherosclerotic plaque development [106].

With its high metabolic activity and the lipid-rich environment to which the brain is exposed, it is singularly vulnerable to oxidative stress concerning neuroprotection. Antioxidant enzymatic components protect neuronal cells from damage by oxidative stress and hence diminish the chances of neurodegenerative disorders such as Parkinson's or Alzheimer's disease. Animal studies indicate that supplementation with these enzymes improves cognitive performance and reduces neuroinflammation. The second critical component of diabetes treatment involves understanding the role of oxidative stress in the pathogenesis of diabetes and its complications, such as diabetic retinopathy and diabetic nephropathy. Other mechanisms of enhancing insulin sensitivity and protection of pancreatic β-cells from oxidative damage, including antioxidant enzymatic constituents, may also be involved in reducing the risk of diabetes complications. Clinical studies have demonstrated the potential of such enzymes to improve glycemic control and reduce markers of oxidative stress among diabetic patients [107]. Chronic oxidative stress can lead to DNA damage and promote carcinogenesis, thus playing a crucial role in cancer prevention and therapy. Antioxidant enzymatic components protect cells from oxidative DNA damage, potentially reducing the risk of cancer. Additionally, these enzymes can enhance the efficacy of cancer treatments by providing resistance against oxidative damage caused by radiation and chemotherapy, thereby protecting normal cells [108].

Maintaining skin health exposes the skin to many forms of oxidative stress including UV radiation, pollution, and inflammation. Protecting skin cells from the damaging consequences of oxidative stress is mostly dependent on antioxidant enzymes, thereby maybe lowering the incidence of wrinkles, photoaging, and even skin cancer. These enzymes have shown encouraging effects in enhancing skin conditions by lowering inflammation and hastening the healing process when included in topical treatments. Maintaining the potency of antioxidant enzymatic components throughout production and standardizing will help to guarantee their usefulness in therapeutic uses. The manufacturing process begins with the cultivation of probiotic strains in controlled environments to promote enzyme synthesis. Subsequently, bacterial cells are harvested from the growth media, and the enzymatic components in the supernatant are removed [109]. Apart from this, standardization includes the quantification of key bioactive compounds besides establishing mechanisms of quality control concerning the stability and potency of such compounds. Highly advanced methods of analysis, such as HPLC, mass spectrometry, and NMR spectroscopy, are usually applied to determine the composition of the antioxidant enzymatic components and to ensure consistency between batches. Safety and regulatory considerations when using antioxidant enzymatic components as postbiotics also play important roles along the line [92]. These products, considering they are manufactured by bacterial fermentation, become highly essential to be free from dangerous contaminants such as endotoxins, mycotoxins, and residual bacterial cells. That calls for strict purification and quality control processes to ensure that such products meet the required safety standards for human consumption. Moreover, the regulatory frameworks for postbiotics, including antioxidant enzymatic components, are still in development. Regulatory bodies such as the FDA and EFSA are currently working on standards and recommendations for the evaluation and approval of postbiotic products. Consequently, these recommendations will likely address concerns regarding safety, effectiveness, labeling, and claims, serving as the foundation for the commercialization of antioxidant enzymatic components [110].

Some of the future directions of research on these areas will involve identifying specific bioactive compounds responsible for the health benefits associated with antioxidant enzymatic components as postbiotics; developing personalized approaches to postbiotic supplementation; and incorporating such components into functional foods and beverages. This would allow the tailoring of postbiotic therapy for the needs of the individual patient, enabled by technological advances in microbiome analysis and biomarker identification. It is also possible to deliver the health benefits of the antioxidant enzymatic components to a large number of people practically and pleasantly through the development of functional foods and beverages that contain the components [111]. Antioxidant enzymatic components hold significant promise as postbiotics, and current research continues to explore their potential uses as well as the mechanisms through which they exert their effects. One area of interest is the identification of specific bioactive compounds found in the supernatants, which are responsible for the health benefits associated with these substances. This insight has the potential to lead to the creation of postbiotic products that are more specifically targeted and effective. Within the realm of customized therapy, the use of supernatants is yet another intriguing option. Personalized methods of postbiotic supplementation might potentially improve their effectiveness, given the individual heterogeneity that exists in the makeup of the gut microbiota and the metabolic reactions that it elicits [15, 112].

This development in microbiome profiling and biomarker identification should consequently enable the tailoring of supernatant-based medicines to meet individual needs. Oxidative stress is at the core of several severe cardiovascular conditions, including atherosclerosis, hypertension, and heart failure. Antioxidant enzymatic components may protect against cardiovascular events by reducing oxidative damage in both the vessels and tissue of the heart. Several studies have looked at the ability of these enzymes to enhance endothelial cell function, reduce lipid peroxidation, and impede atherosclerotic plaque formation. The brain is under very high metabolic activity and in a lipid-rich environment, hence it is particularly vulnerable to oxidative stress [113]. Antioxidative enzymatic constituents can protect neuronal cells against these oxidative stress-related injuries, with implications for lower risk of neurodegenerative diseases such as Parkinson's and Alzheimer's. Animal studies have, in addition, demonstrated that supplementation with these enzymes enhances cognitive performance and diminishes neuroinflammation. The role of oxidative stress in the pathogenesis of diabetes, as well as in associated complications such as diabetic retinopathy and diabetic nephropathy, is a critical factor in diabetes therapy. On the other hand, antioxidant enzymatic components may positively influence insulin sensitivity, protect pancreatic β-cells from oxidative damage, and reduce the risk of diabetes-related complications. Experiments under clinical conditions have already shown that these enzymes can improve glycemic control and reduce indices of oxidative stress in diabetic patients [114].

This may be one mechanism by which persistent oxidative stress promotes carcinogenesis and DNA damage, both of which are very critical in cancer prevention and treatment. Antioxidant enzymatic components, in theory, may protect the cells from the noxious effect of oxidative DNA, thereby probably reducing the risk of tumorigenesis. These enzymes may further enhance the effectiveness of cancer treatment by protecting normal cells from oxidative damage caused by radiation and chemotherapy. The skin is exposed to various oxidative stresses that affect its health, including UV radiation, pollution, and inflammation. In this way, enzymatic antioxidants help protect skin cells from the harmful effects of oxidative stress, reducing the risk of wrinkle formation, photoaging, and even skin cancer. Indeed, topically applied products containing these enzymes have shown the potential to improve skin health by reducing inflammation and accelerating the healing process [115].

Exopolysaccharides (EPSs)

Exopolysaccharides, now more commonly referred to as EPSs, are long-chain polysaccharides excreted into the environment by microbes like bacteria, yeasts, and algae. Their production is extracellular; that is, it occurs outside the microbial cell. They may be attached to the surface of the cell or secreted into the surrounding environment. EPSs have gained much interest in recent years due to the health-beneficial properties they possess, most of which relate to their action as postbiotics. Postbiotics were defined as bioactive compounds produced by probiotics either through fermentation or metabolism [116]. These continue to show therapeutic effects on the host in nature even after bacteria have lost their ability to survive. Other postbiotics, EPSs also find wide applications in medicine, health, and the food preparation industry. Considering their chemical composition and structure, the function of EPSs can vary widely. These EPSs consist of various types of sugars, including glucose, galactose, rhamnose, mannose, and, occasionally, non-sugar components such as proteins or lipids. The presence of this diverse range of components influences the nature and properties of the EPS molecules. These include a wide variety of bacteria responsible for the production of EPS, namely LAB such as *Lactobacillus*, *Streptococcus*, and *Bifidobacterium* species [117]. Food industries often use these bacteria during the manufacturing of fermented foods. In the food business, one of the most important processes is the fermentation of dairy products, and this cannot be said to be complete without the generation of EPSs by probiotics, especially lactic acid bacteria. In addition to enhancing the health benefits associated with probiotics, EPSs improve the texture, viscosity, and shelf life of fermented foods (Table 9). Probiotics are widely recognized for supporting improved health, and in recent years, there has been growing interest in their potential therapeutic applications, including anti-inflammatory, immunomodulatory, antioxidant, and antibacterial activities. These EPSs have possibilities for use in functional foods, nutraceuticals, and medicinal goods because of their qualities. One of the key areas of action for postbiotics is the gastrointestinal system, where there are several positive effects of EPSs [118].

Table 9. Applications of EPSs in health and industry

Application Field	Function of EPSs	Examples	Benefits	Challenges
Food Industry	Improves texture, viscosity, shelf-life	Yogurt, cheese, fermented beverages	Enhanced product quality, consumer satisfaction	Standardizing production methods
Medicine	Modulates immune response, anti-inflammatory	Functional foods, therapeutic formulations	Prevents chronic diseases, supports immunity	Limited clinical trials on specific EPS types
Pharmaceuticals	Drug delivery, wound healing	Encapsulation systems, hydrogel dressings	Controlled drug release, enhanced bioavailability	Ensuring biocompatibility
Cosmetics	Moisturizing, anti-aging effects	Skin creams, anti-wrinkle formulations	Healthier skin, reduced signs of aging	Stability in cosmetic formulations
Environmental Science	Biofilm formation, bioremediation	Wastewater treatment, soil conditioners	Eco-friendly solutions, pollutant breakdown	Cost-effective production at scale

EPSs influence gut health by altering the gut microbiota, strengthening the intestinal barrier, and fostering the proliferation of beneficial bacteria while inhibiting pathogenic development. They may facilitate the formation of short-chain fatty acids in the gastrointestinal tract. SCFAs possess anti-inflammatory properties and are essential for preserving intestinal homeostasis. Butyrate, acetate, and propionate, among the SCFAs, possess these qualities in addition to modulating immune responses, inhibiting colon cancer, and promoting overall gut health. The primary mechanisms through which EPSs exert their therapeutic benefits include interactions with the immune system [119]. In this context, EPSs may modify immune responses by stimulating cytokine production, enhancing the activity of immune cells such as macrophages and dendritic cells, and promoting antibody formation. Due to their immunomodulatory properties, EPSs are useful in conditions deemed to be associated with immunological malfunction. Such diseases include infections, autoimmune diseases, and allergies. Besides that, various EPSs have shown the ability to prevent infectious diseases by blocking the adhesion of pathogens to epithelial cells [120].

The anti-inflammatory properties of EPSs are most relevant for the control of chronic inflammatory diseases, including IBD and IBS. Indeed, several studies have demonstrated that EPSs could block the activation of pro-inflammatory pathways in the stomach or reduce levels of proinflammatory cytokines produced in the gut. It improves overall health in the stomach and intestines through reduced inflammation. Besides anti-inflammatory activity, antioxidant activities of EPSs were reported. Such activity might help protect cells from the damaging actions of oxidative stress and reduce the risk of chronic conditions such as cancer and heart disease. Some research has also been conducted regarding the application of EPSs as an antimicrobial agent. Several studies have evidenced that some types of EPSs exhibit antimicrobial activities against a wide range of pathogens, including bacteria, fungi, and viruses [121]. Antimicrobial effects of EPSs are believed to be a result of interference with the growth and adhesion of pathogens, and their ability to enhance the production of AMPs by the host's immune system. These features make EPSs attractive candidates for applications in infection prevention and treatment, especially in the context of rising antibiotic resistance, which has become a significant public health concern. Another area of EPS research involves their role in enhancing the bioavailability and stability of bioactive substances. Encapsulation by EPSs creates a protective environment for these compounds, shielding them from gastrointestinal degradation and enabling their controlled release at targeted sites of action. This property is particularly useful in drug delivery systems and the development of functional foods designed to provide specific health benefits to targeted patient groups. Since EPSs can form hydrogels, emulsions, and films, they are suited for a wide range of uses in the pharmaceutical and food fields [122].

Besides health-related applications, there are many EPS applications in the industry. Because of gelling, thickening, and stabilizing properties, EPSs find extensive use in the food industry for the improvement of texture and consistency in items like yogurt, cheese, and sauces. Other applications of EPSs are in the cosmetic industries, where it is highly valued for its moisturizing and skin-protective properties. The application of EPSs in the pharmaceutical industry extends to the preparation of drug delivery systems and materials for wound treatment. Due to their biocompatibility, biodegradability, and non-toxicity, EPSs are suitable for a wide range of applications across various industries [123, 124].

Several factors can affect the production of EPSs, which may include the type of microbe, growth medium constitution, and environmental conditions such as temperature, pH, and oxygen level. In industrial settings, optimization of such elements is highly relevant to ensuring maximum output of the EPSs. Recent advances in biotechnology including genetic engineering and fermentation technology, now allow large-scale production of EPSs with features that can be designed according to the necessities of a particular application. For example, by using genetic engineering, one can change the composition of extracellular polysaccharides to improve their functional properties [125]. Examples include enhancing their antioxidant or immunomodulatory activities. In addition to their natural formation through the involvement of microorganisms, synthetic versions can also be obtained using chemical methods. Synthetic EPSs can be designed and fabricated to mimic natural ones in both structure and function, with the added advantage of being tailor-made for specific applications. However, the synthesis process for synthetic EPSs is generally more expensive and less environmentally friendly compared to the production of microbiological EPSs. This may explain why the application of natural EPS remains the best option in most industries. Many studies have been done to determine whether the use of EPSs is safe as postbiotics or not [126].

The conclusion derived is that they are generally regarded as safe for food and pharmaceutical products. Conversely, the efficacy and safety of some EPSs may be origin, composition, and application-dependent. In light of this fact, it is of the utmost importance to carry out rigorous testing to ensure the safety of consumption and health benefits provision capability of EPS-based products. Although there is great encouragement for the possibility of having postbiotics as EPSs, several issues are still to be resolved. One of the main problems that has to be overcome is the heterogeneity regarding the content and structure of EPSs produced by different microbes [127]. This may ensure that products whose base is EPS will be affected regarding their consistency and reproducibility, hence it will be difficult to standardize the production and application of such products. Secondly, further research is needed both to understand fully the mechanisms through which EPSs exert their health-promoting effects and to identify which components of EPSs are responsible for those effects. Full comprehension of such mechanisms is very important [128].

Products of Cell Wall Fragments and Bacterial Lysates

Two forms of postbiotics are produced as a consequence of the breakdown of bacterial cells. These postbiotics include cell wall fragments and bacterial lysates. The breakdown of bacterial cells may occur either naturally or intentionally. These components are generally acknowledged for their capacity to bestow health advantages without the requirement for live bacteria, making them a reliable and risk-free alternative to the conventional probiotics that are currently available. The potential therapeutic uses of postbiotics, produced from bacterial lysates and cell wall fragments, have garnered significant attention from researchers in the fields of science and medicine. In particular, postbiotics have been investigated for their ability to modulate the immune system, improve gut health, and protect against infections [129]. Bacterial lysates are complex mixtures of bacterial cellular components, such as proteins, peptidoglycans, LPS, nucleic acids, and other fragments derived from the microbial cell. Additionally, bacterial lysates may contain other fragments as well. Typically, these lysates are produced by causing the bacterial cell membrane to be disrupted by the use of mechanical, enzymatic, or chemical procedures. To liberate the contents of the intracellular space, the cell wall is broken down by the use of mechanical disruption techniques such as high-pressure homogenization and sonication [130] (Table 10).

Table 10. Therapeutic effects of postbiotic components from cell wall fragments

Postbiotic Component	Source	Immune Mechanism	Therapeutic Effects	Potential Applications
Peptidoglycans	Gram-positive bacterial cell walls	Activates macrophages and dendritic cells	Enhances innate immunity, reduces inflammation	Vaccines, immune-boosting supplements
Lipoteichoic Acids	Gram-positive bacterial lysates	Modulates cytokine production	Decreases pro-inflammatory responses	Treatment for autoimmune disorders
Lipopolysaccharides (LPS)	Gram-negative bacterial fragments	Stimulates antimicrobial peptide production	Fights bacterial infections	Development of infection-resistant drugs
Exopolysaccharides	Fermentation by Lactobacillus and Bifidobacterium	Enhances gut barrier, promotes beneficial microbiota	Prevents leaky gut syndrome, supports gut homeostasis	Gastrointestinal therapies

In enzymatic lysis, the enzymes used, such as lysozyme, degrade the peptidoglycans in the bacterial cell wall. Alternatively, this may be done by using chemical lysis, in which detergents or other chemical agents degrade the cell membrane. It would be possible that the lysate will be of variable composition, given that various kinds of lysis were used, and can give rise to various biological consequences. In contrast, cell wall fragments are specific entities of the bacterial cell wall. They are largely composed of peptidoglycans, teichoic acids, and other structural molecules [90, 131]. These components can be produced either through bacterial lysis or by specific extraction techniques. An example of such essential components in the bacterial cell wall is peptidoglycans. These mainly consist of sugars and amino acids, which play a critical role in maintaining the structure of the cell intact. Teichoic acids are an additional component that imparts rigidity to the cell wall of Gram-positive bacteria. Teichoic acids are present in Gram-positive bacteria. The fact that these fragments are especially well-recognized for their capacity to modulate immune responses makes them helpful in therapeutic applications [132].

A primary advantage of using postbiotic cell wall fragments and bacterial lysates is their ability to regulate the immune system. Numerous studies have demonstrated that these postbiotics can enhance both innate and adaptive immune responses. As a result, they significantly improve immune system function and offer protection against infections. Furthermore, peptidoglycans, which are components of bacterial cell walls, have been shown to activate immune cells, including macrophages, dendritic cells, and neutrophils. These immune cells utilize pattern recognition receptors (PRRs), such as Toll-like receptors (TLRs) and NOD-like receptors (NLRs), to detect peptidoglycans. Due to this identification, a chain reaction of immune responses takes place with the final result of the formation of cytokines along with other immune mediators. These mediators, in turn, help the body in its defense against all types of infections [133]. Moreover, bacterial lysates have been extensively studied for their immunomodulatory properties. One of the most well-known applications of bacterial lysates in immunotherapy is the development of immunostimulatory drugs for respiratory infections. By enhancing the immune system, products like OM-85, a bacterial lysate derived from multiple strains of respiratory pathogens, have been shown to reduce the incidence and severity of respiratory tract infections. OM-85 stimulates the activity of macrophages, dendritic cells, and lymphocytes, thereby contributing to a faster and more robust immune response against infections [134]. This drug has illustrated the therapeutic potential of bacterial lysates by its application in clinical practice for the prevention of episodes of recurrent respiratory infections in children and adults. Another important application of bacterial lysates and cell wall fragments is due to their health-promoting properties in the digestive tract system [135].

The gastrointestinal tract of humans is host to a huge population of microorganisms. In general, these bacteria are known as gut microbiota and play an important role in health maintenance and disease prevention. The gut microbiota can be modulated by the use of postbiotics resulting from bacterial lysates and cell wall fragments. These postbiotics can stimulate the growth of beneficial bacteria and inhibit the proliferation of harmful pathogens, thereby enhancing gut barrier function, reducing inflammation, and improving the synthesis of SCFA-critical events that help maintain gut health. Apart from modulating gut microbiota, it has been emphasized that postbiotics derived from cell wall fragments and bacterial lysates have the potential to improve the integrity of the intestinal barrier [136].

It is an essential defensive system that fulfills the important role of keeping hazardous substances, such as infections and poisons, out of circulation. Breakdown of this barrier may lead to diseases such as leaky gut syndrome, associated with a variety of autoimmune diseases and inflammatory disorders. It has also been shown that bacterial lysates and cell wall fragments may induce the production of tight junction proteins, maintaining the intestinal barrier function. In this regard, postbiotics might help prevent gut permeability and minimize the risk of systemic inflammation owing to the reinforcement of the intestinal barrier. Most of the research has also focused on antiinflammatory activities developed by the postbiotics produced by bacterial lysates and cell wall fragments [137]. Chronic inflammation is widely recognized for its crucial role in the pathogenesis of various diseases, including IBD, IBS, and autoimmune conditions. Several studies have shown that postbiotics, particularly those derived from the cell walls of Gram-positive bacteria, can inhibit the activation of inflammatory pathways and reduce the production of pro-inflammatory cytokines. It has been shown, for example, that peptidoglycans and teichoic acids produced by *Lactobacillus* spp. are capable of inhibiting the activation of nuclear factor kappa B (NF-κB) necessary for regulating inflammation. In that they act on the suppression of NF-κB activation, these postbiotics may have anti-inflammatory action in the prevention of inflammation and symptoms in individuals confronted with chronic inflammatory disorders [138].

In addition, bacterial lysates and cell wall fractions have been able to exert antimicrobial activity, thus becoming beneficial tools in the prevention of infections. Some postbiotics can inhibit the growth of harmful bacteria, fungi, and viruses by directly compromising the integrity of microbial cell membranes or interfering with the ability of these microbes to replicate. The most interesting of these is the LPS, which can be extracted from some bacterial lysates and induce the production of AMPs like defensins, which are important actors in the innate immunological defense of the body. These peptides kill pathogens or prevent infections through their cytolytic action on the cell membranes of the pathogens. Due to their antimicrobial properties, postbiotics derived from bacterial lysates and cell wall fragments are highly valuable for infection prevention, particularly in environments with extensive antibiotic use [130]. In addition to their health benefits, these postbiotics could also find applications in the food and pharmaceutical industries. Because of the antimicrobial properties that they possess, postbiotics could be useful in the food business as a natural preservative. They are capable of prolonging the shelf life of food products by preventing the growth of organisms responsible for foodborne disease and spoilage. Moreover, due to the anti-inflammatory and immunomodulatory properties of these postbiotics, they can be considered perfect candidates for functional foods designed to enhance immunological health with reduced inflammation [111].

Lysates of several bacteria and fragments of their cell wall currently are under study for pharmaceutical application in drug delivery systems. Because they interact with immune cells and affect immunological responses, they become interesting candidates for further development in immunotherapies and vaccines. Certain bacterial lysates, for instance, are employed as adjuvants, substances that enhance the body's immune response to vaccines. The goal of their use would be to bring about an improvement in vaccine efficacy. This application is very promising and holds potential in enhancing the effectiveness of vaccines, particularly in immunocompromised hosts, including elderly adults and those with compromised immune systems [139]. Despite the high and promising potential of postbiotics formed from bacterial lysates and cell wall fragments, many obstacles remain to be overcome. One of the most critical issues is the variability in the composition of bacterial lysates, as it may affect the consistency and reproducibility of the results. The exact composition of bacterial lysates can vary depending on the bacterial strain used, the nature of the lysis method employed, and the conditions present during bacterial growth [140].

This is because bacterial lysates are complex mixtures of cellular components. The diversity that can occur means that differences in biological effects produced by the lysates will be realized, and that presents difficulty in standardizing production and usage for such lysates. Moreover, the detailed mechanisms by which cell wall fragments and bacterial lysates exert their positive effects need to be further investigated for a complete understanding. Although several studies have established the immunomodulatory, anti-inflammatory, and antimicrobial properties of these postbiotics, the exact molecular mechanisms involved in these processes remain to be fully explored. Indeed, a comprehensive understanding of these processes will be crucial for the effective and safe utilization of postbiotics in therapy [141].

Short-Chain Fatty Acids (SCFAs)

SCFAs represent one class of postbiotics, and during the last decade, the major role played by these in human health maintenance has attracted a great deal of attention concerning the regulation of immune response and gut health. The production of SCFAs is driven by the gut microbiota through the fermentation of dietary fibers. These SCFAs include acetate, propionate, and butyrate, which are the most common types of SCFA and for which most studies have been conducted. Besides supplying a source of energy to colonocytes, these bioactive molecules play an important role in the regulation of numerous physiological processes [142]. Besides their local effects on the colon, the fact that they are present in the stomach, circulation, and other tissues brings to light the fact that they have a systemic influence on human health. Dietary fibers resistant to digestion in the small intestine enter the colon, where they are fermented by good gut bacteria, especially those from the genus *Bifidobacterium* and *Lactobacillus*. This leads to the formation of short-chain fatty acids or SCFAs in the large intestine. The fermented products of these bacteria are responsible for the production of short-chain fatty acids, which degrade complex carbohydrates, oligosaccharides, and other prebiotic fibers. This is due to the relative production of acetate, propionate, and butyrate, which depends on the type of fibers fermented and the composition of gut bacteria. For example, it has been estimated that in the colon, approximately sixty percent of the produced SCFAs are acetates. Propionate and butyrate follow in second and third place, respectively, each contributing around twenty percent of the total SCFAs [143].

A critical balance of these short-chain fatty acids is important to achieve optimum health, especially in a functional gut. One of the major functions that SCFAs represent is serving as a source of energy for the colonocytes, the cells lining the colon. Of all the saturated fatty acids, SCFAs, butyrate is particularly important in that it supplies these cells with as much as 70 percent of the energy they require. It is of utmost importance that the epithelium barrier limits the passage of injurious bacteria and toxins from the stomach into circulation, and this energy source contributes to maintaining the integrity of the epithelial barrier. Butyrate also promotes mucus production by goblet cells, further strengthening this protective barrier. A robust epithelial barrier reduces the risk of inflammation and infection, contributing to overall gut health. Given its role in enhancing barrier function, butyrate has become an important target for medications designed to treat and prevent disorders such as IBD and leaky gut syndrome [144].

SCFAs moreover exert systemic effects through their regulation of metabolic, immunological, and inflammatory pathways beyond their local activities in the gut. Short-chain fatty acids, particularly butyrate, have been shown to exhibit anti-inflammatory properties. These compounds exert an inhibiting action on NF-κB, a transcription factor involved in the regulation of inflammatory reactions. This suppression decreased the expression levels of pro-inflammatory cytokines, namely tumor necrosis factors (TNF-α), IL-6, and IL-1β. SCFAs have the possible potency of helping in the management of chronic inflammation, associated with a wide range of ailments including metabolic disorders, cardiovascular diseases, and autoimmune diseases, since they inhibit the production of these cytokines. SCFAs also play a major role in the process of immunological regulation. They influence both the innate and the adaptive immune systems. In the innate immune system, SCFAs enhance the capabilities of macrophages, neutrophils, and dendritic cells [142, 145].

These cells are important in the early defense against infection. For example, butyrate has been shown to enhance the phagocytic ability of macrophages by allowing the cells to more effectively engulf and remove invading bacteria. The defensins are a type of induced antimicrobial peptide, and their production is a result of SCFA stimulation. These peptides target and kill pathogenic microorganisms directly. Due to their presence, SCFAs influence the development and function of T cells, primarily regulatory T cells, which are a part of the adaptive immune system.

Table 11. Detailed functional postbiotic classification

Postbiotic Type	Source	Bioactive Components	Primary Functions	Potential Applications
Short-chain Fatty Acids (SCFAs)	Fermentation of dietary fibers in the colon	Acetate, propionate, butyrate	Enhances gut barrier, regulates inflammation, and provides energy to colonocytes	Treatment of IBD, metabolic syndrome
Exopolysaccharides (EPSs)	Probiotic bacteria like *Lactobacillus* spp.	Glucose, galactose, mannose polymers	Supports microbiota balance, boosts immune function, prevents pathogen adhesion	Food stabilizers, therapeutic drugs for autoimmune diseases
Cell Wall Fragments	*Lactobacillus* spp., Gram-positive bacteria	Peptidoglycans, teichoic acids	Modulates immune response and enhances intestinal barrier	Immunotherapy, vaccines, anti-inflammatory drugs
Bacterial Lysates	Mechanically or enzymatically lysed bacteria	Proteins, DNA, lipopolysaccharides (LPS), enzymes	Stimulates immune cells, reduces respiratory and gastrointestinal infections	Immunostimulatory drugs, vaccine adjuvants
Antioxidant Enzymes	*Lactobacillus, Bifidobacterium* spp.	SOD, CAT, GPx	Neutralizes oxidative stress, reduces chronic inflammation	Cardiovascular health, neurodegenerative disease prevention, skincare

Regulatory T cells are a crucial cell subpopulation involved in maintaining immunological tolerance and restricting excessive immune responses that could lead to autoimmunity [146]. By promoting Tregs differentiation, SCFAs facilitate the prevention of autoimmune responses and the maintenance of immunological homeostasis. SCFAs participate in the gut-brain axis, commonly referred to as the communication from gut to brain (Table 11). This is another important function of SCFAs. The available studies so far would seem to indicate that SCFAs are capable of influencing brain functions and behaviors by several mechanisms [147].

For instance, SCFAs may easily pass the blood-brain barrier to influence neurotransmitter synthesis, such as serotonin, which is involved in mood regulation, appetite, and sleep. It has also been illustrated that short-chain fatty acids, or SCFAs, may reduce neuroinflammation by lessening the production of pro-inflammatory cytokines within the brain. Due to this neuroprotective effect, SCFAs have become of growing interest as therapeutic agents in neurological disorders, ranging from anxiety and depression to neurodegenerative diseases like Parkinson's and Alzheimer's. SCFAs thus modulate glucose and lipid metabolism and, therefore, are also contributors to metabolic health. Specifically, the two- and three-carbon SCFA, namely acetate and propionate, have been shown to have the ability to regulate glucose and lipid production in the liver [148]. Propionate is a substrate for gluconeogenesis, while acetate plays a role in the lipogenic pathway. It has been shown that these SCFAs inhibit cholesterol production in the liver and favor its excretion. Further, there is evidence of a link between SCFAs and improved insulin sensitivity of the key determinants of the development and management of type 2 diabetes. Since SCFAs can regulate metabolism, they have been one of the hot topics in research on obesity and metabolic syndrome. The goal of this study is to design therapies that take advantage of the beneficial effects of SCFAs on energy balance and fat storage [149].

One of the effects of SCFAs is their capability to regulate appetite and the amount eaten. SCFAs are capable of promoting the secretion of GLP-1 and PYY gut hormones. These two hormones are very important in suppressing appetite and producing a feeling of satiety. SCFAs stimulate the secretion of these anorectic hormones, thus regulating food intake and preventing overconsumption of food for the maintenance of body weight. Reduction of appetite by SCFAs was demonstrated in various animal and human studies. This makes SCFAs a potential candidate for formulating dietary strategies in the prevention and treatment of obesity. Although there are numerous health benefits associated with SCFAs, their composition and production may vary due to several factors, including diet, gut microbiota composition, and overall health status. The diet should include sufficient amounts of fiber-rich foods, such as fruits, vegetables, whole grains, and legumes, to support SCFA production. Specific gut bacteria ferment different types of fiber—primarily soluble fibers like inulin and resistant starches—into short-chain fatty acids [150].

For example, the butyrate-producing bacteria, such as *Faecalibacterium prausnitzii* and *Eubacterium rectale*, can grow best on resistant starches and nondigestible polysaccharides, thus leading to an increased production of butyrate. In contrast, for a diet with low fiber and including more processed foods and fats, SCFA production is significantly decreased, the balance of microbiota in the gut is disrupted, and the impacts on health become negative. Another major determinant that affects the output of SCFA is the bacterial composition within the gut tissue itself. Having a healthy and diverse microbiota is highly necessary for the proper fermentation of dietary fibers and the production of SCFAs [151]. Dysbiosis refers to an imbalance in the gut microbiota that may decrease the synthesis of SCFA and increase the number of pathogenic bacteria. That has been associated with several health conditions, such as abnormalities in the gastrointestinal tract, obesity, and inflammatory diseases. Treatment by diet, probiotics, or prebiotics may restore dysbiosis and increase the synthesis of SCFA, which could be associated with an improvement in general health. Recent research has also focused on the medicinal value of SCFAs in disease treatment and prevention. IBDs are disorders wherein the gastrointestinal tract remains inflamed for a period longer than is typical for any normal inflammatory process [152].

Examples of IBD include Crohn's disease and ulcerative colitis. There is some evidence to suggest that short-chain fatty acids, specifically butyrate, may help improve symptoms of IBD by reducing inflammation, restoring the epithelial barrier, and enhancing mucosal healing. Clinical studies have defined that butyrate supplementation, or probiotics capable of producing butyrate, may decrease disease activity and increase the quality of life in patients with IBD [153]. Further, SCFAs have been studied to understand their potential role in cancer prevention, particularly in colorectal cancer. Butyrate has been shown to induce programmed cell death in neoplastic cells, suppress tumor formation, and stimulate the differentiation of normal colonic epithelium. Based on these findings, the use of this agent as an anti-tumor agent has been pursued. Even as SCFAs have been associated with various health benefits, such challenges must be overcome before these findings can be translated into actual therapeutic applications that could be used in the real world. This may be one of the difficulties faced by the industry: there are many variables, including genetic makeup and environmental and lifestyle factors, that affect the heterogeneity of SCFA production. Moreover, whereas SCFAs are typically considered harmless, their impact may be contingent on the quantity being provided or under conditions in which they have been administered. For example, overproduction of SCFAs, especially acetate, has been associated with adverse metabolic outcomes, including fat storage and insulin resistance. Thus, to maximize the health benefits of SCFA supplementation or nutritional interventions while at the same time minimizing the potential risks, there may be a need for personalization in these treatments [154].

Chapter 6

Postbiotic Preparation Techniques

Abstract

This chapter focuses on the various techniques used to prepare postbiotics, outlining the main steps involved in their synthesis and isolation. The production of postbiotics starts with fermentation, where probiotic bacteria are cultured under specific conditions to generate bioactive metabolites. The chapter provides an in-depth discussion on fermentation parameters, bacterial lysis methods, and the extraction and purification of postbiotics. Special attention is given to the role of enriched media in optimizing the yield of bioactive compounds. Methods for the isolation and characterization of postbiotics, including SCFAs, peptides, and polysaccharides, are detailed, alongside the challenges and innovations in improving postbiotic production. The chapter concludes by discussing the scalability of postbiotic preparation for industrial applications.

Introduction

These procedures span a range of postbiotic preparation methods to extract and concentrate the existing bioactive chemicals in bacterial cultures. For this reason, such approaches have become essential because of the production of postbiotics capable of providing therapeutic and health advantages devoid of the use of live bacteria. The components that make up the postbiotics involve inactivated bacterial cells, pieces of cell walls, metabolic products, and any other elements that may have been beneficial for one's health. Each form of preparation has a procedure and objectives peculiar to it while the chosen route of preparation is somewhat responsible for its overall quality and effectiveness [140]. Fermentation is a process in the preparation of postbiotics where the culture of probiotic bacteria is maintained under controlled conditions for the generation of bioactive compounds. The selection of appropriate strains of probiotics would be the first step in the whole process and would involve organisms such as

Lactobacillus, *Bifidobacterium*, or *S. boulardii* since all these have been identified to confer positive benefits.

The Main Steps in Postbiotic Synthesis

After strain selection, the growth of this strain is carried out in a medium that provides all the necessary growth requirements, primarily nutrients and optimal conditions. In postbiotic manufacturing, key parameters to consider include pH, temperature, and oxygen levels. Other examples of bioactive compounds synthesized during the bacterial fermentation process include short-chain fatty acids, antimicrobial peptides (AMPs), and various other metabolic compounds. These kinds of compounds are produced due to the metabolic action of the bacterium on the substrate available in the medium [155, 156].

Fermentation Conditions

There are limited ways that fermentation can be carried out, such as batch, fed-batch, and continuous fermentation, based on the conclusion to be attained. After the fermentation process is completed, the bacterial culture is harvested and the postbiotics in the supernatant are extracted. This usually involves separating the bacterial biomass from the liquid phase, where the postbiotics dissolve. Centrifugation and filtration are among the various methods used for such separations. Next follows purification and concentration. Contraction methods, including evaporation or ultrafiltration, reduce the volume of supernatant while concentrating the postbiotics. Further steps of purification may then be done based on different chromatographic techniques, where some of the postbiotics are separated and contaminants eliminated [157].

Bacterial Lysis

Another commonly used method is bacterial lysis, based on the disruption of bacterial cells to release their intracellular content and fragments of the cell wall. Bacteria may be lysed using mechanical disruption, enzymatic lysis, and chemical lysis. The mechanical disruption techniques include high-pressure homogenization and bead milling, where physical pressures are used to rupture the bacterial cell walls. The process of high-pressure homogenization forces the bacterial solution through a tight space, where cells undergo very high pressure that causes the breaking of the cell walls. Bead milling relies on the mechanical agitation of the bacterial culture in the presence of abrasive beads, which causes the crushing of cells. Sonication is a process that applies sound waves to generate shear pressures that break the cells of bacteria [158]. Enzymatic lysis involves the degradation of several parts of the bacterial cell wall due to the action of specific enzymes. For example, lysozyme will cleave peptidoglycans in Gram-positive bacteria cell walls. Because of this specificity and controlled action, enzymatic lysis is usually done since it has the potential to assist in maintaining the integrity of the postbiotics that are in demand. Chemical lysis can break the membranes surrounding bacterial cells using chemical agents such as detergents or solvents. Certain detergents, like SDS and Triton X-100, can dissolve cell membranes and release the constituents inside the cell. While chemical lysis is effective, it must be handled carefully to avoid unwanted chemical residues in the final product [159].

Extraction and Purification

After the bacterial cells had been lysed, the resulting mixture was made up of pieces of cell wall, among other cell components. These pieces may undergo further processing to extract and purify certain postbiotics. The separation and purification of the compounds needed are typically carried out by various techniques, including centrifugation, filtration, and chromatography. Bacterial lysis produces specific compounds, such as cell wall fragments, which contain peptidoglycans and teichoic acids, due to their immunomodulatory activity. Through the various steps in the preparation of postbiotics from fragments of cell walls, the lysate is often further purified to achieve these components in their isolated form. Techniques that could be employed for this include gel filtration chromatography and ion exchange chromatography [160]. The metabolites produced due to bacterial fermentation are another important category of postbiotics. In this category, bacterial lysates and cell wall fragments will be included. Moreover, such metabolites, which are usually present in the culture supernatant, need to be concentrated and purified. Some examples of such metabolites are SCFAs.

Approaches such as solvent extraction, membrane filtering, and chromatographic procedures are only some of the many different approaches to this [161]. Solvent extraction involves adding a solvent that selectively dissolves the target metabolites, and then further separating those metabolites from the aqueous phase. After this, evaporation of the solvent leaves much more concentrated metabolites. Filtration techniques of ultrafiltration and nanofiltration have been applied to effect the separation of metabolites according to their molecular weight. These techniques make use of membranes of very precisely defined pore diameters. Chromatographic techniques such as HPLC and Gas Chromatography (GC) are used in further purifying and analyzing the metabolites [162].

Enriched Medium

Other than fermentation, another method for producing postbiotics is by fermentation with prebiotics, which includes the simultaneous addition of prebiotic fibers in the process. Prebiotics are carbohydrates that are indigestible but have the property of selectively stimulating the growth of some beneficial bacteria in the stomach. Since postbiotics are composed of SCFAs and other metabolic products, these can be possibly produced with the aid of prebiotics because this will provide an additional substrate for fermentation [163]. It may be that the production and composition of postbiotics can be improved using prebiotics in fermentation to make postbiotics more useful for applications in health. Following development, postbiotics are usually compounded into various formulation forms, differing in their application and distribution. Examples of this include powders, capsules, pills, and liquid formulations. The type of formulation chosen is based on the application intended for the postbiotic and the stability criteria needed. While nutritional supplements are usually manufactured in powdered or capsule form, functional foods or beverages may use liquid formulations [164].

Another step-in formulation involves the stabilization of the postbiotics to ensure efficacy and prolong the shelf life of the metabolites. This could involve excipients, preservatives, and methods of encapsulation. Since environmental factors, such as temperature, humidity, and light, may affect the functionality of postbiotics, stability represents an important issue that has to be considered during the development process of postbiotic ingredients. The application of stabilization procedures protects the postbiotics against degradation and also tries to maintain their bioactivity. Encapsulation is a technique where postbiotics are either coated or embedded in a protecting coating/matrix that protects them from various external factors and allows gradual release utilizing a process. This will enhance the stability and controlled release of the postbiotics, hence being more effective in health applications [165].

Chapter 7

Safety Assessment of Postbiotics

Abstract

Ensuring the safety of postbiotics is critical for their widespread use in both therapeutic and food products. This chapter discusses the various safety assessment protocols required for postbiotics, including toxicity testing, immunogenicity evaluation, and the establishment of safety profiles. The chapter examines the importance of strain selection and fermentation conditions to minimize the risk of contaminants and harmful by-products. Additionally, the safety of postbiotics in vulnerable populations, such as infants, elderly individuals, and immunocompromised patients, is explored. Regulatory guidelines for the approval of postbiotic products are also reviewed, emphasizing the need for rigorous clinical trials to confirm their safety and efficacy. The chapter concludes by discussing the future directions in postbiotic safety assessment and regulatory frameworks.

Safety Profile of Postbiotics

Safety assessment in the setting of health and disease management is, thus, a critical process that constitutes the very foundation upon which the utilization of postbiotics is based. Indeed, postbiotics are a fast-emerging area of interest, considering the bioactive compounds including inactivated bacterial cells, cell wall fragments, and microbial metabolic products potential therapeutic benefits. However, before these products are allowed for human consumption or application, a critical review ought to be carried out to ascertain whether they are safe or not. Such reviews are supposed to take into consideration various factors that relate to manufacturing processes, characterization, possible dangers, as well as regulatory issues [166]. First, the manufacturing process of postbiotics is an area very closely related to the safety of these specific ingredients. First, the selection of appropriate bacterial strains should take place. Those should be sufficiently described by relevant health authorities, and their status needs to be ascertained about their

GRAS status. The selection of appropriate strains is of paramount importance because the use of pathogenic or dangerous strains could pose serious risks to human health. High consideration is given to strains that are well-recognized for their positive benefits without pathogenicity. Bacterial strains are selected for postbiotic production and then cultivated under precisely calculated conditions. Culture medium, temperature, pH, and oxygen levels are carefully and systematically controlled to achieve the highest possible level of bioactive chemical synthesis. This approach helps prevent the formation of unwanted impurities or by-products when the parameters are maintained at optimal levels. For instance, if the fermentation process is not properly managed, it could lead to the growth of undesired microorganisms or the production of harmful chemicals that may negatively impact the ecosystem [167].

The next process after fermentation is rendering the bacterial cells inactive. This is quite an important process in that it ensures the bacteria are no longer alive, hence removing any kind of danger associated with the presence of living germs. Other approaches used to inactivate them include heat treatment, irradiation, or chemical intervention. Each method has its advantages and possible disadvantages. For instance, heat treatment can effectively kill bacteria but can also destroy some useful components of postbiotics. On the other hand, chemical methods can include residues that one should manage with care. Afterward, postbiotics are extracted from the culture medium. This typically involves the separation of the bacterial biomass from the supernatant, wherein the postbiotics will be present [168]. Centrifugation and filtering are some of the various techniques used for this separation. Then, the supernatant is filtered for concentration and purification to separate postbiotics of interest. Concentration methods applied in increasing the concentration of postbiotics include evaporation and ultrafiltration. On the other hand, chromatography is one of the purification techniques used to remove impurities and isolate specific molecules. Characterization is a critical process in the safety assessment of postbiotics. For one to confirm that the postbiotics are indeed what they claim to be, there is the need to identify and measure components that make up postbiotic material. To accomplish the aforementioned, a range of analytical techniques such as HPLC, mass spectrometry, and NMR are typically applied. By fully characterizing postbiotics, one can confirm the composition of postbiotics and ensure that postbiotics do not contain unexpected or toxic compounds. In addition, it's important to know about the study of the biological action of postbiotic bacteria [169, 170].

Toxicity Assessment

Their impact, therefore, on cellular activities, immunological responses, and metabolic processes is an integral part of the assessment process. It is also important that if postbiotics can modulate the immune system or affect gut health, it is indicated to confirm its supposed effects. In this respect, all unexpected or adverse outcomes must be revealed for the sake of postbiotic safety. The most crucial types of safety examination involve toxicity testing. Based on this study, it will be confirmed whether postbiotics possess the ability to harm cellular and tissue frameworks in humans [63]. Toxicity assessment often involves an array of in vitro assays employing cell lines and in vivo studies using animal models. This is done to establish any potential hazard and to ensure that postbiotics, upon administration in the intended manner, do not cause any adverse effects. Care will have to be taken with the list of potential hazards that come with postbiotics. Some individuals have questioned its potential allergic reactions. It is highly unlikely that persons are allergic to some ingredients of postbiotics, such as proteins or polysaccharides, at times. Allergy testing and monitoring will be required for the discovery and treatment of the allergic reactions that may conceivably occur. However, the other important factor is immunogenicity. For instance, it might well be that those postbiotics produced from bacterial cell walls or even fragments could have immunogenic properties that may lead to an unintended response of the immune system [171].

Immunogenicity

Investigations into immunogenicity are rewarding in that they provide useful insights into whether or not postbiotics may have the ability to cause inflammatory or hypersensitive responses. It is essential to ensure that the use of postbiotics does not lead to the development of any adverse immunological responses. Another significant concern at present is contamination. Monitoring the manufacturing process is necessary to prevent contamination with potentially hazardous microorganisms or chemical residues. The tests needed to check against microbial pollutants like pathogenic bacteria or fungi are so essential to assure cleanliness in postbiotic goods. These include tests for any potential contaminants that could have been generated either during fermentation itself or in handling. One more area of concern is the interaction with various medications.

Indeed, postbiotics have the potential to modify the efficacy and safety profile when taken with some medications [116]. The interaction studies are quite fundamental in the full understanding of how postbiotics could influence medication metabolism and treatment effects. This helps ensure that the postbiotics will not interfere with the efficacy of drugs given while at the same time preventing undesirable effects from taking place. When determining whether postbiotics are safe or not for use, regulatory concerns remain quite an important factor. While most regulatory frameworks in the world require proof of both safety and efficacy for postbiotics to be approved for application, it may change from region to region. This includes preclinical study data, clinical trial data, and post-market surveillance information. The regulatory authority ensures that postbiotics are accurately labeled regarding their composition and any claimed health effects, and that all required safety conditions are met. Proper quality control is essential for compliance with regulations [172].

Safety Establishment in the Manufacturing Scale

The manufacturing process for postbiotic products should be uniform and must fulfill all the needs concerning safety. Manufacturing must, to the letter, follow Good Manufacturing Practices that ensure postbiotics are manufactured under conditions that preserve their quality and safety. Routine testing for contaminants and quality control protocols are among the most relevant features that ensure safety in postbiotic products. Looking into the future, there are a series of topics that will take prominence in research and development in the field of postbiotic safety evaluation. Long-term studies are required to understand the chronic effects and long-term health impacts of postbiotics. Personalized safety profiles may help in the identification of postbiotic use tailored to the needs of an individual based on genetic, environmental, and health-related variables. This will ensure the safety and efficacy of postbiotics, as it will improve the accuracy and reliability of safety assessments through the development of new technologies for pollutant and bioactivity detection [173].

Chapter 8

Potential Bio-Utilization of Postbiotics

Abstract

This chapter explores the bio-utilization of postbiotics in various therapeutic applications, focusing on their role in modulating metabolism, promoting wound healing, and supporting immune functions. Postbiotics, particularly short-chain fatty acids (SCFAs), are discussed for their ability to enhance metabolic processes and reduce the risk of atherosclerosis, obesity, and other metabolic diseases. The chapter also highlights the detoxification and wound-healing properties of postbiotics, detailing their role in tissue regeneration and infection prevention. Furthermore, the chapter examines the potential of postbiotics in functional food formulations and their antibacterial effects. The applications of postbiotics in treating gastrointestinal, neurological, and immunological infections are also considered, with a focus on their bioactive components.

Immunomodulation and Anti-Cancer Effects

In recent years, postbiotics have gained the limelight in health research due to their potential applications in immunomodulation and anti-cancer therapies. Besides possessing functionalities that include those of live probiotics, the bioactive ingredients formed by inactivated bacterial cells, cell wall fragments, and microbial metabolic products present a variety of benefits not accessible with live probiotics. Since postbiotics, in contrast with living microorganisms, do not require active living bacteria to act, they are a very useful subject of research because of the therapeutic potential they carry. One of the most important fields wherein postbiotics have shown their potential is immunomodulation [174]. The immune system is a complex network of cells and proteins that helps defend the body against infectious agents and can be influenced by various factors, including postbiotics. These compounds can interact with immune cells in several ways, affecting their function and activity. For example, postbiotics have been found to exert an immunomodulatory effect on macrophages, which are key immune cells responsible for pathogen phagocytosis and antigen presentation to other immune cells. By enhancing macrophage activity, postbiotics may also improve the body's ability to combat infections [175].

Postbiotics may act not only on macrophages but also on other immune cells, such as dendritic cells and T and B cells of the immune system. Postbiotics could influence dendritic cells, which are the cell types responsible for the initiation of immunological reactions, in this respect. Their effect can enhance the ability of dendritic cells to stimulate T cells. This could enhance the immune response and make it more specific. Another possibility is the effect of postbiotics on cytokine production so-called signaling molecules that are responsible for the regulation of immunological responses. Postbiotics, as one of the probiotic metabolites, can help balance inflammatory responses by modulating cytokine production. This can eventually help in reducing chronic inflammation and diseases associated with the condition. Another key area of postbiotics relates to their impacts on gut microbiota, which is very crucial in the regulation of immune function [176]. Diversity among gut bacteria is the hallmark of gut microbiota, which interacts extensively with the immune system through different angles. The gut microbiota composition can be modulated by the use of postbiotics, and it might reinforce the growth of helpful bacteria while impeding harmful bacteria. Given that GALT is a major portion of the immune system, this can eventually enhance gut health and improve immunological function [177].

Besides the immunomodulation capabilities, postbiotics have the potential to be extended in cancer treatment and prevention. Currently, postbiotics are being explored for anti-cancer potentials, of which several mechanisms are under investigation. One-way postbiotics may help in treating cancer is through improvement in the recognition capability of the immune system for destroying cancerous cells. It can enhance immune cells, including T cells and macrophages, which play critical roles in decision-making processes regarding the choice between attacking tumor cells and recognizing them (Figure 1).

This may enable postbiotics, through immune modulation, to contribute to controlling tumor growth and improving patient outcomes [178]. Another possibility is that postbiotics exert their influence on cancer via the induction of apoptosis kind of programmed cell death. Apoptosis is one such natural mechanism that helps eliminate defective or damaged cells through the active process of cell death.

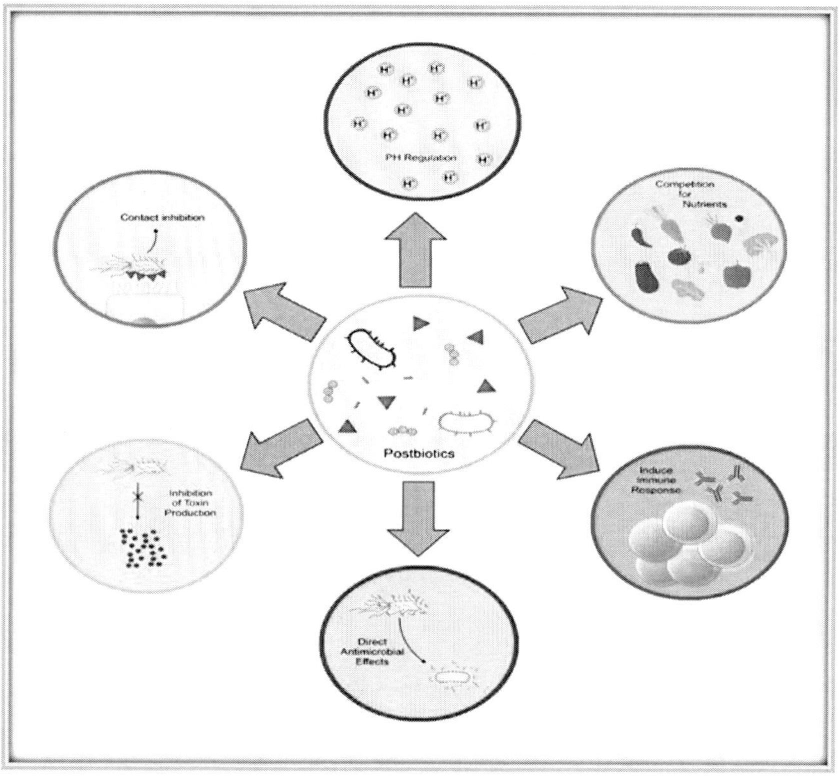

Figure 1. Potential mechanisms of effect of postbiotics.

Abnormal regulation of apoptosis might lead to the development of tumors. It has been demonstrated that some postbiotics can induce apoptosis in tumor cells without affecting normal cells, thus eliminating the tumor cells. It is thus envisioned that this selective induction of cell death may be beneficial in reducing tumor burden and preventing cancer proliferation [90]. Additionally, postbiotics can help prevent tumor development through a variety of mechanisms. For instance, some postbiotics may have the potential to hinder processes such as angiogenesis, the formation of new blood vessels that supply a tumor. They appear to slow down tumor growth and the spread of metastases due to reduced angiogenesis. Diverse postbiotics can exert direct effects on the proliferation of tumor cells, hence acting as retardants to tumor growth. Further research is still ongoing to identify specific postbiotics and the effect they elicit on immunomodulation and cancer [175].

Other research has been conducted on postbiotics obtained from different strains of probiotics, like *Bifidobacterium* and *Lactobacillus*. Those studies have been reported as promising, and some postbiotics are showing potential for enhancing immune responses and inhibiting the proliferation of cancer cells in preclinical models. In contrast, despite this fact, more research, particularly clinical trials, will be needed to fully realize such capabilities of postbiotics and also to prove their effectiveness and safety in clinical settings in human populations. Consideration needs to be made to the awareness that postbiotics will be ingested as therapeutic agents due to the potential benefits they could confer in immunomodulation settings and cancer therapies [179]. It is also crucial that further research in this field continues relentlessly, focusing on studying the modes of action, improving production and application, and conducting appropriate clinical testing of efficacy. According to ongoing studies, postbiotics could become valuable tools in combating neoplastic diseases and enhancing immune function. This would provide new opportunities for their application in developing countries, ultimately improving health outcomes [180].

Metabolism Modulation and Anti-Atherosclerotic Effects

In recent times, postbiotics have gained considerable attention as an interesting family of molecules in health and disease management due to their association with metabolic control and anti-atherosclerotic action. Due to this fact, those bioactive substances, including inactivated bacterial cells, cell wall fragments, and microbial metabolites, have quite substantial potential to influence various physiological processes without the presence of living microorganisms. This property makes postbiotics very desirable in the development of treatment methods for metabolic disorders and cardiovascular illnesses [13]. The study of the influence of postbiotics on metabolic processes belongs to the area of vast studies. Metabolism is a term used to describe biochemical changes taking place in living organisms for life support. These activities include conversion of food into energy, elaboration of cellular structures, and maintenance of a range of physiological activities. These postbiotics can affect glucose homeostasis, lipid metabolism, and even the amount of energy being expended by the body. Another important method of interaction between the postbiotics and glucose metabolism involves interaction with bacteria that reside in the gut [181].

The gut microbiota is a complex bacterial community inhabiting the digestive system and plays an important role in glucose homeostasis. Postbiotics, a derivative of fermented probiotics, might induce changes in the composition and activity of the gut microbiota, which could be one of the contributors to enhanced insulin sensitivity and glucose uptake. SCFAs, such as acetate, propionate, and butyrate, for example, are known to be produced by gut bacteria via fermentation. It is also widely acknowledged that these SCFAs influence the pathways in insulin signaling [164]. These SCFAs, therefore, help improve insulin sensitivity to maintain blood sugar within normal limits, thereby decreasing the risk of insulin resistance and even type 2 diabetes. On top of all these, postbiotics have the potential to influence gene expression linked with glucose metabolism. With the possibility of modulating enzymes and transcription factors involved in glucose homeostasis, postbiotics could favor proper metabolic functions. The fact that such control could be useful in preventing metabolic pathologies such as diabetes underlines how important it is to gain information about detailed mechanisms through which postbiotics might have the ability to alter glucose metabolism [182].

Other essential areas where the effects of postbiotics can be observed involve lipid metabolism. Some of the lipids involved in lipid metabolism include cholesterol and triglycerides. The catabolism and transportation of lipids are also under lipid metabolism. The disturbance in lipid metabolism can lead to a condition known as hyperlipidemia, which involves the elevation of lipid levels in the blood. Hyperlipidemia is among the most important risk factors that predispose humans to cardiovascular illness. Postbiotics may alter lipid production and breakdown in the liver and other tissues throughout the body, thereby changing lipid profiles [183]. They may also decrease the circulating levels of Low-Density Lipoprotein (LDL) cholesterol and increase those of High-Density Lipoprotein (HDL) cholesterol, which is considered to have positive implications for cardiovascular health. The postbiotic action on gut microbiota is one common mechanism of action to how these metabolites play their role in lipid metabolism. Postbiotics exert their effectiveness in altering the absorption and metabolism of lipids by promoting the proliferation of beneficial bacteria while suppressing the growth of harmful bacteria. Additionally, the gut microbiota synthesizes short-chain fatty acids (SCFAs), which play a role in regulating gene expression during lipid synthesis and storage. This regulation of the lipid profile may help prevent atherosclerosis, which is characterized by plaque buildup in the arterial walls, thereby reducing the risk of related complications [184].

Another target of action regarding metabolism on which postbiotic food supplements may act is the expenditure of energy. We use the term energy expenditure to describe the amount of energy taken up by the body. It is an important parameter when it comes to the prevention of obesity and maintenance of weight. Indeed, postbiotics may influence energy expenditure through their effects on metabolic rate and thermogenesis [185]. A few studies have shown evidence that postbiotics can enhance the activity of brown adipose tissue (BAT), a specific type of fat tissue implicated in the generation of heat and oxidation of fat. Increased BAT protein activities are suggested to present the potential of postbiotics in enhancing weight management and reduction of obesity risk. The anti-atherosclerotic properties of postbiotics are closely related to their influence on metabolism [186]. Atherosclerosis is a chronic inflammatory disease characterized by the deposition of plaques in the arterial walls, leading to reduced blood flow and increased risk of cardiovascular events, including heart attacks and strokes. Postbiotics have thus shown efficacy in several ways for the prevention and management of atherosclerosis. Of the major factors leading to atherosclerosis, chronic inflammation plays a leading role. In this regard, postbiotics may reduce inflammation by changing the immune response that affects the production of pro-inflammatory cytokines. An example is that certain postbiotics inhibit the activation of nuclear factor-kappa B, a transcription factor responsible for genes governing inflammation. Hence, this kind of postbiotics reduces inflammation and, in turn, promotes cardiovascular health by inhibiting the onset of atherosclerosis [187].

Aside from the fact that postbiotics confer anti-inflammatory properties, they also have the potential to affect lipid profiles and thus may play a vital role in atherosclerosis prevention. Improvement in lipid profiles may inhibit the formation of plaques in arteries and reduce the risk of cardiovascular diseases by reducing LDL cholesterol among others and raising the level of HDL cholesterol. Further, the modification of lipid metabolism by postbiotics may involve the control of genes linked to cholesterol metabolism and transport, thus supporting cardiovascular health. The other key component of cardiovascular health that may be improved by the use of postbiotics includes endothelial function [88]. The endothelium is a thin layer of cells that lines blood vessels, and its proper functioning is crucial for maintaining the vascular system in a healthy state. Indeed, postbiotics exert an effect that improves endothelial function by enhancing the production of nitric oxide (NO), a chemical mediator involved in the regulation of blood vessel dilation and the reduction of oxidative stress. By improving endothelial function, atherosclerosis can be prevented and general cardiovascular health supported, helping to avoid the development of diabetes. Research into the metabolic and anti-atherosclerotic activities of postbiotics is still in its infancy, but several studies have thrown up encouraging results [188].

Postbiotics from various probiotic strains have been demonstrated to improve glucose metabolism, lipid profiles, and endothelial function in animal models and early human studies. However, a complete understanding of the modes of action whereby postbiotics act requires further research, as does determining the safety and efficacy of postbiotics in human subjects. Challenges faced in this industry are many, among them standardized postbiotic products to ensure consistency concerning their quality and effectiveness. Also, more studies should be conducted to identify the real postbiotics and specific responses by various metabolic pathways on vascular health. There is, therefore, a further need for the development of the technique of analysis and a full understanding of the postbiotic processes involved in developing appropriate postbiotic-based therapies for metabolic diseases and atherosclerosis [172].

Detoxification and Wound Healing Effects

Some of the interesting molecules with great potential in several therapeutic areas, including detoxification and treatment of wounds, are postbiotics. These bioactive components-inactivated bacterial cells, cell wall fragments, and microbial metabolic components-can act outside the presence of a live microorganism and therefore confer advantages complementary to those provided by live probiotics. For the complete exploitation of postbiotics' therapeutic potential, a thorough understanding of the role they play in detoxification processes and the process of wound healing has to be present [189]. Detoxification has been defined as the process by which the body removes toxicants or inactivates them. It is an important physiological function in health maintenance and the prevention of disease. Through a variety of avenues, postbiotics have shown potential to improve detoxification processes. Among the important avenues through which postbiotics might contribute to the detoxification process, influencing gut microbiota stands prominent [190]. The gut microbiota forms an important part of the metabolism and excretion of toxins. Postbiotics can modulate gut microbiota composition and activity to complement this role. For instance, postbiotics may affect the production of short-chain fatty acids, the metabolic end-products of bacterial digestion of food fibers in the stomach. It is well established that SCFAs, including acetate, propionate, and butyrate, are involved in gut health maintenance and the promotion of toxin elimination. Postbiotics may contribute to the enhancement of detoxification and excretion capability in the gut through modification of the production levels of short-chain fatty acids [191].

Besides influencing gut microbiota, postbiotics may interact with the liver, considered the most important blood-purifying organ. The liver processes a great variety of toxins by enzymatic reactions into neutral substances; this could also be enhanced by postbiotics. It has been documented that some postbiotics can affect the activity of liver enzymes and, consequently, may enhance its capacity in the detoxification and excretion processes of various harmful chemicals. The relevance of such an effect is particularly significant under conditions of impaired liver function or when exposed to environmental pollutants. Additionally, postbiotics may help reduce oxidative stress, which is characterized by an imbalance between the generation of reactive oxygen species (ROS) and the body's ability to neutralize them [192]. The result of oxidative stress could be cell and tissue damage, and it might contribute to many disorders. Antioxidant postbiotics may inhibit ROS and therefore decrease oxidative stress, leading to an improvement in detoxification processes. Wound healing is another domain in which postbiotics have shown promise as beneficial [193].

It is a very complex process that comprises inflammation, the creation of new tissue, and the remodeling of pre-existing tissue. Until now, postbiotics have indicated the capability to affect more than one phase in wound healing, specifically: regulation of the inflammatory response, stimulation of repair processes in the tissues, and cellular regeneration. Generally, postbiotics regulate inflammation and, as such, are one of the ways they contribute to wound healing [194]. While inflammation forms an important phase in wound healing, on the contrary, excessive or long-term inflammation may impede the process and give rise to problems. For example, postbiotics could exert anti-inflammatory activity via modulation of the inflammatory response by influencing the production of cytokines or other inflammatory mediators. Some postbiotics have been reported to decrease the levels of pro-inflammatory cytokines, such as TNF-α and interleukin-6. This might subsequently contribute to preventing excessive inflammation and could support a healing process. Another possibility is that postbiotics stimulate tissue repair by modifying the activity of a variety of cells that participate in the wound-healing process [195]. For example, fibroblasts are crucial cells involved in the production of collagen and other extracellular matrix components essential for tissue repair. It has been noted that some postbiotics promote fibroblast proliferation and increase collagen production, both of which can accelerate the wound healing process [196].

Apart from postbiotic involvement in the regulation of inflammation and healing of tissues, there is cellular regeneration. Cellular regeneration plays a major role in the healing of tissues following injury, as well as in general tissue health. Besides, postbiotics may influence the cellular events of proliferation, differentiation, and apoptosis, each important for proper wound healing. Therefore, due to the stimulation of cellular generation, postbiotics can enhance the healing rates of wounds and thus the outcomes of wound management. Further research is ongoing to examine such effects of postbiotic influence on detoxification and wound healing.

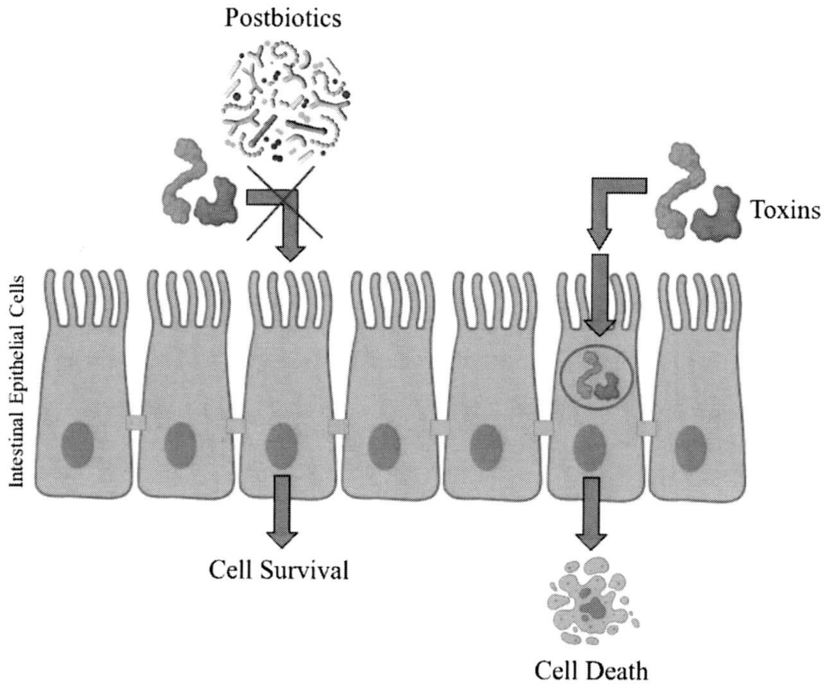

Figure 2. Mechanism of toxin inhibition through postbiotics.

Although several promising results have been published, further research will be needed fully to understand the modes of action and the therapeutic possibilities of postbiotics. Which postbiotics are involved and what effect they have on detoxification and wound healing will depend, among others, on the origin of the postbiotics, the postbiotic composition, and the environment in which they are used [197] (Figure 2).

Functional Food Preparation

During the formulation of functional foods, postbiotics are becoming one of the important ingredients as they contribute highly to the health-promoting attributes of such food. Contrarily, postbiotics are the bioactive molecules of either bacterial cell or metabolic by-product origin. These include inactivated bacterial cells, cell wall fragments, and microbial metabolites. Active probiotics are live microorganisms that have gained increased attention due to their potential benefits in gut health, metabolic function, and immune support, among other areas. Their role in functional foods has become a growing focus [198]. Functional foods are defined as foods that, in addition to providing basic nutrition, offer health benefits. These foods can prevent disease, treat existing conditions, and improve overall health, thereby enhancing the quality of life. One of the emerging approaches to adding value to functional foods is the incorporation of postbiotics. This approach confers specific health benefits without the use of viable microbes. One of the most interesting areas in functional food development involves gut health, within which the evolution of postbiotics takes part. That refers to populations of different bacteria living inside the digestive system that form what is called the gut microbiota, very vital for sustaining proper digestive health and general well-being [199]. Postbiotics may have a positive influence on microbiota through modification of its composition and activity. A proper gut microbiota might be developed; the growth of beneficial bacteria might be improved, and the proliferation of pathogenic microorganisms hindered just by the addition of postbiotics to functional foods. The generation of SCFAs is one of the most important ways postbiotics influence the maintenance of gut flora [200].

SCFAs are produced by the fermentation of dietary fibers through gut bacteria. They mainly include butyrate, propionate, and acetate. The main roles of SCFAs are to supply energy for intestinal cells, contribute to the integrity of gut barriers, and possess anti-inflammatory functions. The latter might enhance SCFA synthesis, therefore contributing to a better digestive tract in promoting gut health. In addition to the impact on SCFAs, postbiotics may affect gut mucosal immunity [201]. Postbiotics could act on the modulation of immunological activities by interacting with gut-associated lymphoid tissue, GALT, which plays an important role in the immune response of the body. This interaction could be of critical importance in building barriers that protect the stomach from harmful invaders, reducing inflammation, and enhancing general immunological function. This might be better supported, and these immune responses enhanced, by the inclusion of postbiotics in functional meals at a higher level. A second key area of concern is the possibility that postbiotics will have a significant effect on metabolic function. The metabolic process involves biochemical processes responsible for converting food into energy and controls a range of physiological activities. A variety of metabolic processes, including glucose metabolism, lipid metabolism, and energy expenditure, are susceptible to the influence of postbiotics [202].

Considering their influences on insulin sensitivity and glucose absorption, postbiotics may modulate glucose metabolism. It has been showed that various postbiotics produced from fermented probiotics could improve insulin sensitivity. This is because insulin sensitivity has a significant role in blood sugar regulation and, consequently, the prevention of metabolic disorders such as type 2 diabetes. This effect is often mediated by changes in gut microbiota composition and the production of SCFAs, which may influence insulin signaling pathways and significantly improve glucose metabolism. In addition to glucose metabolism, postbiotics may also impact lipid metabolism [203]. An imbalance in lipid metabolism can lead to conditions such as hyperlipidemia and cardiovascular disorders. Indeed, postbiotics can affect the lipid profile by altering the synthesis and degradation of lipids. Given this potential, postbiotics could lower LDL cholesterol levels and increase HDL cholesterol levels. This process of lipid metabolism modulation is beneficial to cardiovascular health and can therefore contribute to the prevention of atherosclerosis. Another metabolic aspect that postbiotics may influence in nutritional supplements is energy expenditure [204]. With postbiotics, the rate of metabolism and thermogenesis can be affected, hence, may help in weight management and decrease obesity. According to various other studies, the postbiotics also may activate brown adipose tissue that generally participates in heat production and fat oxidation. Having this effect could help improve energy expenditure and thus support the maintenance of a healthy body weight [88].

Postbiotics represent formulas that, besides affecting gut health and metabolic function, strengthen the immune system. The latter represents a multi-component system of cells, tissues, and organs working together to protect the body from all sorts of diseases and infections. It is the task of the immune system to protect against diseases. Accordingly, the postbiotics may have several functions for the immune system: modulation of inflammation, enhancement of immunological response, and improvement of immune function generally. Of these, one of the primary ways in which postbiotics alter immunological tissue function is through their ability to modulate inflammation [205]. Whereas inflammation is an essential component of the immune response, excessive or chronic inflammation can lead to a variety of health disorders of varying severity. Given their ability to modulate the production of pro-inflammatory cytokines and other mediators, postbiotics may play a role in regulating inflammation [206]. It has been demonstrated that some postbiotics can reduce the levels of specific cytokines, such as TNF-alpha and IL-6. The application of such postbiotics could help prevent excessive inflammation, promoting a balanced immune response. The postbiotics may interact directly with immune cells or tissues and may, therefore, enhance immunological responses. In this way, they could help the body's resistance against infection and illness by modulating the activities of immune cells like macrophages, dendritic cells, and T cells. Such immune responses could be enhanced, and general immunological health supported, by the inclusion of postbiotics in functional meals. Since the postbiotics are to be incorporated into the preparation of functional foods, their origin, content, and stability have to be approached with care [207].

Different postbiotics will have different effects, based on their origin and method of preparation. Those postbiotics, for example, that come from specific probiotic strains could impart health benefits different from those others emanating from other sources. Moreover, stability during the preparation of food and storage is considered the most important factor in identifying the usefulness of postbiotics in functional meals. For that reason, standardization of postbiotic products would be fundamental to ensuring constant quality and efficacy. This involves the discovery and measurement of bioactive components, besides the development of optimal delivery strategies that preserve the stability and activity of these components [208]. Where maximizing the inclusion of postbiotics into functional meals is involved, advances in analytical techniques and formulation methods become highly essential. With postbiotics having a promising future in functional foods, several issues are yet to be resolved. Further research is needed to understand the mechanisms by which postbiotics exert their activities and also to establish the safety and efficacy of postbiotics in various uses. Clinical research in this respect is highly demanded to confirm both the health benefits of postbiotics and the best usage of these substances in functional food [209].

Antibacterial Effects

It has been increasingly known that postbiotics, bioactive compounds produced either directly by microbes during fermentation or released upon their death, act against bacteria. Such actions have been antibacterial, antiviral, antifungal, and antiparasitic, hence proving a potential for therapeutic uses. Unlike live probiotics, postbiotics offer stability and efficacy without the participation of living microorganisms. For this reason, they are, therefore, a very effective tool in the struggle against various kinds of diseases. Quite remarkably, their antimicrobial activity is widespread, as studies have shown that they combat a wide range of bacterial infections [210]. One of the key mechanisms through which postbiotics exert their antibacterial effects is by playing a crucial role in the generation of antimicrobial peptides (AMPs), which are small peptides produced by bacteria with the ability to inhibit or kill other pathogens. AMPs interact with bacterial cell membranes through their destabilization, hence leading to cell death. The mode of action can operate very effectively against Gram-positive and Gram-negative types of bacteria, among a wide range of bacteria. For example, postbiotics obtained from *Lactobacillus* and *Bifidobacterium* have been reported to be effective against pathogenic bacteria like Escherichia coli and Staphylococcus aureus. The other important trait of the antibacterial activities of postbiotics is their organic acid production potentiality, such as lactic acid and acetic acid, during fermentation [211].

These organic acids increase the acidity of the environment through a drop in its pH, hence creating an acidic situation that is inhibitory to the growth of a large number of bacteria injurious to the health of humans. Another mechanism through which postbiotics may exert an antibacterial action is through the production of hydrogen peroxide. Hydrogen peroxide is a ROS that can lead to the death of bacterial cells through the damaging of cellular DNA, proteins, and lipids. This process has been indicated in various postbiotics generated by LAB [212]. Quorum sensing is a process through which bacteria can communicate with one another and take any particular action based on their population density. This process, too, is affected by the mechanism of postbiotics. These interfere in the quorum sensing process generation of bacterial biofilms, which are detailed communities of bacteria that attach to a surface and are resistant to conventional antibiotics. This capability of disrupting the formation of biofilm is highly useful in the management of chronic infections and impeding the development of bacterial resistance [213-215]. Besides their antibacterial capabilities, it has been found that postbiotics also show potential in antiviral applications. Interference with viral replication or preventing viruses from attaching themselves to host cells is also possible through the action of postbiotics. For instance, some postbiotics, metabolites derived from probiotics, have been observed to exhibit antiviral activity against respiratory viruses such as influenza and coronaviruses. This effect occurs at multiple levels, including the production of antiviral peptides, interference with viral entry, and modulation of the host's immune response [216-218].

There is a connection between the antiviral effects of postbiotics and the influence that they have on the microbiota in the stomach. It is the microbiota that lives in the gut that plays a significant part in the formation of the immune system and in determining how the body reacts to viral infections. Postbiotics can improve the immunological response of the host against viruses by being able to modulate the microbiota in the gut [219]. Postbiotics, for example, can stimulate the production of interferons and other antiviral cytokines, both of which are essential for generating an efficient immune response against viral infections. The use of postbiotics has also been shown to offer promise in the treatment of fungal infections. Postbiotics can exert antifungal effects via a variety of mechanisms, including the generation of antifungal chemicals and the prevention of fungal growth and reproduction. It has been shown that some postbiotics that are produced from bacteria, such as *Lactobacillus* and *Bifidobacterium*, are effective against fungal pathogens, such as *Candida albicans*, which is a frequent source of opportunistic infections. This antifungal effect of postbiotics may entail the rupture of fungal cell membranes, the suppression of ergosterol manufacture which is an essential component of fungal cell membranes, and the interference with the metabolism of fungal cells [220].

An area of study that is only beginning to emerge is the function that postbiotics play in the fight against parasitic infections. Postbiotics can alter parasitic infections by interfering with their life cycle, preventing their proliferation, and modifying the immunological response of the host. For instance, several postbiotics have shown potential in lowering the survivability of parasites like Giardia lamblia and Entamoeba histolytica because of their capacity to inhibit their growth. The methods by which postbiotics exert anti-parasitic effects may include interference with the metabolic activities of the parasites, increase of the immunological responses of the host, and disruption of the relationships between the parasite and the host [111]. The antimicrobial effects of postbiotics comprise a wide range of activities, including antibacterial, antiviral, antifungal, and antiparasitic actions. In general, postbiotics have antimicrobial properties. There are several benefits that these bioactive compounds provide in comparison to live probiotics, including stability, effectiveness, and the simplicity with which they may be included in a variety of formulations. Several postbiotics elicit their antimicrobial action via the generation of different compounds: AMPs, organic acids, hydrogen peroxide, and disruption of quorum sensing [221]. Among other positive effects, postbiotics can alter the composition of gut microbiota, stimulate immune responses, and inhibit the growth and proliferation of harmful microorganisms. As ongoing research continues to reveal their full potential, the use of postbiotics in therapeutic and preventive approaches is expected to increase. Products based on postbiotics may be developed to treat a variety of illnesses and improve overall health outcomes. Further research is necessary to achieve complete elucidation of mechanisms of action and to improve postbiotic formulations, but also to test their therapeutic applicability in many different health situations [217].

Chapter 9

Postbiotics in Medical Bacteriology

Abstract

This chapter examines the therapeutic use of postbiotics in medical bacteriology, focusing on their role in the treatment of various infections. Postbiotics have shown promise in the management of gastrointestinal, urinary, immunological, cutaneous, and neurological infections. The chapter discusses the mechanisms by which postbiotics exert their antibacterial effects, including the inhibition of pathogenic bacteria, modulation of the immune response, and support of the gut barrier function. Specific examples of postbiotics, including cell wall fragments, exopolysaccharides, and short-chain fatty acids, are highlighted for their efficacy in treating infections. The chapter also explores the clinical applications of postbiotics in the treatment of common bacterial infections and their potential as an alternative to conventional antibiotics.

Postbiotics and Gastrointestinal Infections

Diarrhea, stomach discomfort, nausea, and vomiting are the usual manifestations of gastrointestinal infections. Etiology can be caused by anything from very simple bacteria and viruses to fungi and parasites. The traditional approach to treatment normally involves the use of antibiotics and antiviral medications; however, such therapy faces problems in the form of resistance development and the appearance of adverse effects. By directly attacking pathogens and modulating the host's response in a variety of different ways, postbiotics provide a supplementary strategy to the management of these illnesses. One of the major ways through which these postbiotics assist in managing gastrointestinal illnesses is through their antimicrobial action. Antimicrobial chemicals produced by postbiotics, metabolically generated from probiotic strains, can suppress harmful microorganisms [222]. For instance, some strains of *Lactobacillus* and *Bifidobacterium* are capable of forming bacteriocins, which are a type of

AMPs. These peptides can kill off hazardous bacteria like *Clostridium difficile* and *E.coli* on contact by specifically targeting those bacteria. In this way, the peptides lower the pathogen load in the gut by either disrupting bacterial cell membranes or interfering with essential cellular processes [212]. Besides the production of AMPs, the fermentation of postbiotics increases organic acid production, such as lactic acid and acetic acid. By lowering the pH in the gastrointestinal tract, these acids create an acidic environment that inhibits the proliferation of harmful bacteria while promoting the survival of beneficial microorganisms. In addition to preventing the growth of pathogenic bacteria, this acidity helps maintain balance within the gut microbiota [88].

Another important function that postbiotics may play in managing gastrointestinal infections are disruption of biofilm production. Biofilms are complex colonies of bacteria that adhere to surfaces, including the lining of the gut, and that are enveloped in a protective matrix. One factor contributing to the persistence and pathogenicity of infections is that of biofilm creation [223]. Certain postbiotics have been reported to interfere with the quorum sensing method by which bacteria communicate with other bacteria of the same species to signal and coordinate activity, possibly interfering with biofilm creation. For example, it has been determined that postbiotics derived from *Lactobacillus plantarum* can prevent the biofilm formation of pathogens such as Salmonella enterica. Interfering with biofilm formation, postbiotics can increase the efficiency of other treatments and decrease the burrow of infections targeting the gastrointestinal tract. Postbiotics are also of prime importance in the modulation of gut microbiota. The gut microbiota is a heterogeneous bacterial entity that plays a highly essential role in normal digestion, metabolism, and immunological function. A balanced gut microbiota is necessary to keep gastrointestinal health in tune and to avoid infection. Postbiotics may modify the intestinal microbiota composition and activity by promoting the growth of beneficial bacteria while impeding the growth of pathogenic bacteria [208].

This regulation contributes to a healthy gut balance that is important for infection prevention and management. For example, postbiotics can encourage the growth of bacteria responsible for metabolites useful to an individual. Such beneficial metabolites include short-chain fatty acids, which have anti-inflammatory properties and further enhance gut health. Evidence also exists to show that there is a possible use of postbiotics in antiviral applications aside from their antimicrobial effects [163]. This could involve interference with viral replication, inhibition of viral attachment to host cells, and modulation of the immunological response of the host. Some of the postbiotics derived from probiotics have shown antiviral activity against respiratory and gastrointestinal viruses, such as influenza virus, tuberculosis, and norovirus. There are several putative mechanisms by which the observed antiviral activity may be mediated, including the production of antiviral peptides and the maturation of the host immune systems [224-228].

Fungal infections, though rare as compared to bacterial and viral infections, are also treatable with postbiotics. Antifungal chemicals were generated; inhibiting the growth and proliferation of fungi are some mechanisms through which postbiotics may induce an antifungal effect. The postbiotics - metabolic products derived from bacteria - have been shown to exert an effective action against fungal pathogens, such as *C.albicans*, one of the most frequent agents responsible for opportunistic infections. The antifungal action of postbiotics may involve the disruption of fungal cell membranes, inhibition of key biosynthetic pathways, or interference with cell metabolism [229]. The role of postbiotics in combating parasitic infections is a young area of investigation. Indeed, postbiotics can interfere with the life cycle, proliferation, and immunological response against parasitic infections. In the case of parasites such as Giardia lamblia and Entamoeba histolytica, for example, postbiotics have shown that they are capable of weakening them. Among the possible modes of anti-parasitic action of postbiotics, interference with metabolic activity, increasing the immunological responses of the host, and disturbance in the relationships between the parasite and the host may be pointed out. The variety of postbiotic benefits presented to the management of gastrointestinal infections is quite numerous [199].

They are suitable for large formulations such as functional meals and dietary supplement usage due to their high stability rate. Because of their stability, they will be appropriate to use at large scale without refrigeration or sophisticated conditions of storage that they require. Another benefit of postbiotics is that, unlike conventional antibiotics, they have less of a likelihood of inducing antibiotic resistance. This is a result of the fact that postbiotics are manufactured products obtained through bacterial fermentation processes or cellular components [230]. Although postbiotics have shown significant promise, their modes of action require further elucidation to improve the formulation and therapeutic evaluation of these compounds. Clinical trials and research are essential for determining the types and quantities of postbiotics that are most effective against various gastrointestinal diseases. Further research should focus on the identification of which postbiotic strains are most beneficial, developing an understanding of how these strains interact with other members of the gut microbiota, and exploring potential applications of these strains in combination with other therapeutic approaches [231].

Postbiotics and Urinary Infections

Urinary tract infections (UTIs), or - more precisely - infection of the urinary tract is a very common health problem among many people around the world. The most common infective agent responsible for UTIs is *E. coli*; however, other bacteria, such as Klebsiella pneumoniae and Proteus mirabilis, fungi, and viruses can lead to the development of UTIs. Antibiotics are one of the general modes of treatment for UTIs, though this class of drugs has several disadvantages, including the generation of antibiotic resistance, relapsing infection, and disturbing side effects [232, 233]. In the treatment of such diseases, postbiotics could act as an alternative or complementary approach. Antimicrobial potential is one of the significant roles that postbiotics play in the treatment of UTIs. Antimicrobial compounds can be produced from the postbiotics sourced from probiotics strains in a wide variety of ways. These chemicals inhibit injurious bacteria. Examples are bacteriocins, which are produced by certain strains of probiotics and are AMPs. Certain bacteria can select target cells, identify them, and kill them [234]. The production of bacteriocins against some common uropathogens such as E. coli. For instance, it has been realized that postbiotics from strains such as *Lactobacillus* and *Bifidobacterium* are typified by AMPs against *Klebsiella pneumonia*. These peptides act in disrupting membranes within the bacterial cells or interfering with a cellular process of relevance, which consequently leads to a reduction in the number of pathogens that may be present within the urinary tract [235].

Besides bacteriocins, postbiotics generate organic acids, such as lactic and acetic acid, through the process of fermentation. These acids decrease the pH of the urinary surroundings to create an acidic situation. This prevents the growth of a significant number of bacteria harmful to the body, at the same time promoting healthy microorganisms. This acidity can help maintain a healthy microbial flora in the urinary system, preventing the proliferation of bacteria that are harmful to the urinary tract and further promoting its overall health. In urinary infections, interference with biofilm development is another critical point of such pharmaceutical postbiotics.

Inside the urinary tract, biofilms are complicated microbial communities attached to a surface and enveloped by a protective matrix. Biofilms may also reside on surfaces outside the urinary tract [236]. There is a close relationship between biofilm production and the persistence and resistance of infections. By interfering with the mechanisms involved in the attachment of bacteria to surfaces and the formation of biofilms, postbiotics have the potential to disrupt biofilm production. For instance, postbiotics derived from *Lactobacillus* species were reported to suppress *E. coli* from producing a biofilm. This can help reduce the severity of the infection of the urinary tract and could also increase the effectiveness of other treatments [218].

Other roles that postbiotics play include the modulation of microbial ecology that exists within the urinary system. It controls the populations of bacteria to prevent infection. By encouraging the growth of beneficial bacteria and inhibiting the growth of pathogenic germs, postbiotics can influence the composition of the microbial flora. For instance, postbiotics from *Lactobacillus* strains exert an activity that favors the growth of *Lactobacillus* and other beneficial bacteria while inhibiting the growth of uropathogens. The modulation keeps the microbial ecology in a balanced state, which on the other hand reduces the chance of infection. Besides their antibacterial effect, there is some evidence to show that postbiotics may find an application for antiviral purposes. Their presence may interfere with viral replication, inhibit viral attachment to host cells, or modulate the host's immunological response. So far, some postbiotics derived from probiotic strains have been reported to exhibit antiviral activity against viruses in the respiratory and gastrointestinal tracts. However, these postbiotics may also be effective against viruses affecting the prostate. Synthesis of AMPs and maturation of the immunological defenses of the host are two possible mechanisms that might explain the antiviral activity of postbiotics. These mechanisms could be advantageous in the management of viral infections of the urinary tract [237]. Infections caused by fungi may also be treated with postbiotics, even though they are less compared to infections caused by bacteria and viruses. UTIs may be caused by fungal pathogens; for example, Candida species. Immunosuppressed patients are highly susceptible to infection from these diseases. Some postbiotics suppress fungal development and reproduction either by the generation of antifungal chemicals or by the suppression of growth and inhibition of reproduction. The postbiotics produced by some bacterial strains combat fungal infections by inducing perturbations in the cell membranes and interfering with the metabolic functions of fungal cells [238].

One of the most recent fields of study is the role that postbiotics play in fighting parasite infections of the urinary system. Parasite infections of the urinary system are extremely rare compared with bacterial, viral, and fungal infections; however, postbiotics can be useful in conditions if they are provided. They have the potential to control parasitic infection through disruption of their life cycle, inhibition of development, and modulation of the host immune response. For instance, postbiotics have shown that they are capable of reducing the survival of parasites that may cause interference with the urinary system. The potential mechanism for this includes interference with the parasite metabolism and enhancement of the host's immunological response [239]. Postbiotics offer several advantages in the management of urinary infections. They are particularly suitable for large-scale use, as they are typically stable and can be incorporated into various formulations, such as nutritional supplements or functional foods. Another advantage of postbiotics is that they do not require sophisticated preservation or refrigeration. Furthermore, compared to classic antibiotics, postbiotics are less likely to induce resistance in bacteria. This is attributed to their origin from bacterial fermentation processes or cellular elements [240, 241]. However, despite their promising potential, postbiotic modes of action would require further study, enhancement of their formulation, and determination of clinical efficacy. For the complete definition of the types and quantities of postbiotic products effective for the treatment of various urinary infections, clinical trials and research are urgently needed. Further research is required to establish which postbiotic strains are most efficacious, the understanding of how these strains interact with other constituents of the urinary microbiome, and the possible uses of such strains in combination with other modes of treatment [242].

Postbiotics and Respiratory Infections

The future possible therapeutic roles of postbiotics in several types of medical disorders, but with a focus on respiratory infections, have resulted in increased interest in these materials. These bioactive chemicals are produced either by microbes during fermentation or obtained from their cellular content and represent an alternative or supplemental approach to traditional medicine. In contrast to probiotics, postbiotics are generally stable and can exert positive effects even when no active microorganisms are present. Their stability also renders them an excellent drug of choice in the treatment of respiratory infections, a prevalent condition whose treatment is further compromised by various factors such as drug resistance, inadequate efficacy, and adverse effects [243]. Respiratory tract infectious diseases encompass a wide range of symptoms and illnesses, from the common cold to sinusitis, bronchitis, and pneumonia. The etiologic agents of these diseases include bacteria, viruses, fungi, and parasites. Antibiotics, antiviral drugs, antifungal pills, or combinations thereof may be used in pharmacological therapy for respiratory infections [244]. New therapeutic strategies are desperately needed, however, since antibiotic resistance is becoming a serious concern and the current therapies are often unsatisfactory. By focusing on infections, influencing the immune response, and bolstering general respiratory health, postbiotics offer a potentially valuable alternative or complementary strategy. One of the most significant mechanisms of action of postbiotic antimicrobial activity involves mitigation of the growth of pathogenic microorganisms. Accordingly, in postbiotics originating from probiotic strains, the generation of compounds with antimicrobial action could be envisioned. The bacteria of the postbiotics - for example, *Lactobacillus* and *Bifidobacterium* species - may produce bacteriocins. These peptides are antibacterial in action and act against susceptible bacteria. Generally, it leads to a lower bacterial burden on the respiratory tract by the disruption of bacterial cell membranes or interference with some critical cellular functions. The postbiotics can ferment the organic matter to produce bacteriocins and other organic acids such as lactic acid and acetic acid [243].

These acids acidify the respiratory environment by reducing the pH. This acidic environment favors the survival of useful microbes. It inhibits the growth of many pathogenic germs. This acid helps the respiratory microbiome to not get out of balance, which in turn helps in hindering excessive bacterial overgrowth that might be bad for respiratory health. It is vital to maintain this microbial diversity as a gentle balance that keeps away infections. Postbiotics regulate respiratory microbiota through the growth of good bacteria while inhibiting the growth of bad bacteria. For example, research has evidenced that postbiotic metabolites derived from probiotic strains can enhance the proliferation of good bacteria and hinder the dissemination of harmful bacteria. Well-thwarted microbial ecology ensures infection prevention and good general health of the respiratory system. One major reason why lung infections could be so protracted and serious has to do with the development of biofilms [244].

Biofilms are colonies of microbes forming on surfaces and, because they are wrapped in a protective matrix, can better resist treatment. By preventing the mechanisms that bacteria use to attach to surfaces and create biofilms, postbiotics may prevent biofilm development [245]. For instance, it has been shown that postbiotics produced by *Lactobacillus* spp. Prevent biofilm formation of bacteria like *Staphylococcus aureus* and *Pseudomonas aeruginosa.* It forms other treatments more effective by repressing the formation of biofilms. Besides antibacterial action, postbiotics also show anti-viral activity. Respiratory viruses include coronaviruses, influenza, and rhinoviruses [246]. Possible modes of action for postbiotics include modulation of the host immune response, inhibition of virus attachment to host cells, and interference with viral replication. Some postbiotics produced by probiotic strains have demonstrated antiviral activity against respiratory viruses by enhancing host immune defenses and producing antiviral peptides. This could serve as a valuable additional tool in the fight against viral respiratory tract infections. Though less common than bacterial and viral diseases, fungal infections can also affect the respiratory system. For those that are immunocompromised, fungi such as Candida species may also cause infections of the respiratory tract [130].

Postbiotics may have anti-fungal activities on top of the production of anti-fungal chemicals by preventing the growth and reproduction of fungi. In general, the anti-fungal effects of postbiotics from some bacterial strains are manifestations through membrane disruption and interference in metabolic pathways. Respiratory parasite infections seldom occur; however, postbiotics might prove to be helpful even against such infections. They may affect parasitic infection by interfering with the life cycle, dwarfing parasite development, and modulation of the host's immune response. Suppression of the vitality of parasites that can affect the respiratory system through postbiotics shows promise. The anti-parasitic effects of postbiotics may arise from the enhancement of the host's immune response or interference with parasite metabolism [247].

The treatment of respiratory infections by the use of postbiotics has numerous benefits. Because they are relatively stable, their application varies in incredibly many forms, from functional meals and nutritional supplements. They are convenient to use since they do not require special storage or refrigeration conditions. They also pose less threat to antibiotic resistance compared to conventional antibiotics because they source from bacterial fermentation processes or cellular components. While there is every reason to believe that postbiotics may be promising, we still lack sufficient knowledge regarding how best to apply them in a clinical setting, improve formulations, and measure efficacy [243]. Clinical trials and investigations need to be done to find an optimal postbiotic for many respiratory infections. More research is required to find the optimal postbiotic strains, understand those interactions with the remaining respiratory microbiota, and explore their use in concert with other treatment modalities [248]. Finally, in the treatment of respiratory infections, postbiotics stand for armor in weaponry. They hold a wide range of potential benefits due to their antimicrobial, antiviral, antifungal, and anti-parasitic properties. Besides conventional medicine, postbiotics surely promise a very bright future due to their change in microbiome, prevention of biofilm formation, and enhancement in the immunological response of the host. Further research might place postbiotics among the standard therapeutic interventions in respiratory health, with better outcomes and reduced dependency on traditional antibiotics [214].

Postbiotics and Immunological Infections

The immunological infections range from simple conditions to very complicated ones. These are infections where the immune system is either overactive or overwhelmed by the microorganisms to eventually create sickness. Such infections could be from autoimmune diseases, chronic inflammatory syndromes, or states of immunocompromise where the rate of infection is heightened or the virulence is worse. As postbiotics possess the ability to alter immune responses, reduce inflammation, and improve the response of the immune system in general, they bear the potential to be of great service in the treatment of a variety of different diseases. The most significant intervention postbiotics use in the modulation of immunological diseases is the regulation of the immune system. The immune system, a complicated network of substances, cells, and tissues, is involved in protecting the body against infections. The various networks work in concert to defend the body [249]. To enhance the functioning of the immune system or restore homeostasis, postbiotics could interact with many components of the immune system. Some postbiotics have been found to induce the production of cytokines, which are signaling molecules involved in controlling immune physiological responses. Postbiotics from strains of *Lactobacillus* could subtly increase the pro-inflammatory cytokines such as IL-6 and TNF-alpha, thus enhancing the body's response to infections. Moreover, postbiotics can enhance the production of anti-inflammatory cytokines such as IL-10 and thus reduce undue inflammation in a state of excessive inflammation to prevent damage to tissues. Other than the induction of cytokine production, postbiotics may modulate the function of a wide array of immune cells, including T cells, macrophages, and B cells [250].

A good example would be the finding that postbiotics produced by *Bifidobacterium* species have been found to enhance phagocytic activity among macrophages. This plays a very critical role in the engulfing and clearance of infections. Alternatively, it might be that they affect T cell growth and activation positively; in this case, this would raise bodily capacity to fight infections and, as such, would maintain a homeostatic immune response. In fact, through their direct interaction with immune cells, postbiotics help establish an immune system that is proper and timely. A wide range of immunological diseases and autoimmune disorders share a common feature: inflammation. Chronic inflammation can exacerbate symptoms and lead to soft tissue damage [251]. Postbiotics may play a significant role in reducing inflammation by modulating inflammatory pathways, thereby dramatically decreasing the production of pro-inflammatory mediators. Some postbiotics inhibit NF-kB, a transcription factor that regulates genes involved in inflammation. By preventing NF-kB activation, postbiotics lower the levels of inflammatory cytokines and other mediators associated with chronic inflammation. Additionally, postbiotics can influence the activity of inflammatory enzymes such as lipoxygenase and COX-2, further reducing inflammation and its associated effects [252, 253].

It has implications for gut flora, which in turn plays an important role in regulating systemic inflammation. This is apart from the direct effect they may have on inflammatory pathways. The use of postbiotics maintains a healthy gut microbiota by increasing the population of beneficial bacteria without allowing the growth of pathogenic bacteria. This, therefore, enhances systemic immunological balance and reduces inflammation. Besides, postbiotics are of great importance in the context of autoimmune diseases characterized by cases of the immune system attacking tissues of its own body [164]. Regarding autoimmune illnesses, postbiotics can help modulate the immunological responses, thus limiting the excessive quantum of immune activation. They might influence the production of autoantibodies and affect the function of autoreactive T cells in such a manner that could lead to an easing of symptoms from autoimmune diseases. Certain postbiotics, for instance, may modulate the activity of regular T cells responsible for maintaining immunological tolerance and preventing autoimmunity. Apart from immunological regulation and inflammation, postbiotics can improve the barrier capacity of epithelial tissues to maintain general immune health. The epithelial barrier integrity, representing the first line of defense against infection, has to be maintained by an individual if they want to keep off illnesses. Postbiotics may improve the epithelial barrier by inducing the expression of tight junction proteins, thus enhancing the immune response in the mucosal area [254].

An increased barrier function translates to a reduction in the incidence of infections and a decrease in the translocation of pathogens. Although preliminary research has indicated that postbiotics might be considered for use as an adjunctive therapy, studies on postbiotics about immunological disorders are ongoing. Clinical trials are thus needed to fully understand the type and dose of postbiotics that may be most helpful against a range of immunological diseases. Besides an assessment of safety and efficacy across wide ranges of populations, another important finding would be the respective formulations or strains that confer maximum benefits [143].

Postbiotics and Cutaneous Infections

Cutaneous infection is a disorder involving the skin, which is one of the most important barriers against infectious agents. Diseases affecting the skin can be caused by bacteria, fungi, viruses, and parasites; therefore, their care is managed differently for each disease. A few examples of bacterial infections include impetigo and cellulitis, fungal infections that include athlete's foot and ringworm, viral infections that include herpes simplex, and parasitic infections that include scabies have their special problems regarding treatment. One of the main ways in which postbiotics may have an impact on cutaneous infection is a direct effect on the infecting bacteria themselves [230]. Fermentation of bacteria to produce postbiotics can result in AMPs - small proteins that could inhibit infectious bacteria and fungi. One of the most common skin infection-causing pathogens is Staphylococcus aureus. In literature, postbiotics from the species *Lactobacillus*, among others, proved effective against this bacterium [255]. These AMPs interfere with essential cellular processes or disrupt the membrane surrounding the microbial cell, thereby reducing the pathogen's ability to survive and proliferate. In addition to the production of AMPs, postbiotics derived during fermentation can include organic acids such as lactic acid and acetic acid. The presence of these acids lowers the pH of the skin, creating a localized environment that is less favorable to disease-causing microbes while being more supportive of opportunistic beneficial bacteria [256].

The effect of acidification supports the healthy skin microbial flora that leads to reduced incidence of diseases caused by opportunistic pathogens. Apart from the above main aspect, postbiotics involve modulation of immune response in the skin. The skin's immune system is highly involved either in the process of combating an infection or in ensuring that it is healthy. In this regard, postbiotics can affect various levels of the immune response from cytokine production to the activation of immune cells. For example, certain postbiotics are capable of inducing the production of anti-inflammatory cytokines like IL-10, thereby reducing the magnitude of tissue damage and excessive inflammation. It modulates the immune response, therefore enhancing the skin's potential to fight off infections and further support the healing process [180]. Besides, postbiotics influence the function of the skin barrier, an effective way to prevent infections and maintain skin integrity. The skin barrier epithelial cells are tightly joined to one another, thereby forming tight junctions that help prevent the entry of invasive diseases and toxins. Postbiotics have been identified as enhancing overall skin barrier function to improve the production of the proteins contained within the tight junctions. For instance, it has been shown that postbiotics produced by *Bifidobacterium* enhance the expression of occludin and claudin-1-these proteins are important for maintaining epithelial barrier integrity. Improved barrier integrity of skin tissue could reduce infection risk and might be associated with accelerated healing. Antifungal properties of postbiotics have been shown, for example, in fungal infection, which can then be applied in the treatment of various diseases such as athlete's foot and ringworm [221, 257].

It has also been proven that the postbiotics derived from strains like *Lactobacillus* and Saccharomyces inhibit the growth of fungi such as *C. albicans*, which mostly arise from fungal skin infections. Due to the antimicrobial compounds produced by postbiotics that interfere with the membranes or metabolic processes of fungal cells. This leads to alleviated infection burden and better skin health. Other viral cutaneous infections, such as herpes simplex, may be treated by postbiotics, which offer antiviral advantages. Apart from impeding the entry of viruses into host cells, some postbiotics may interfere with the replication of certain viruses. In vitro studies showed that postbiotics obtained from *Lactobacillus* strains can inhibit herpes simplex virus replication [220]. Their action could help with the control of viral infection and reduce symptoms. These changes in the virus's activity, as well as the contribution to the immunological host response, are two ways postbiotics exert their action. It can be used against parasitic diseases such as scabies based on the putative effects on immunological regulation and fortification of the skin barrier. Postbiotics can form the skin barrier to prevent reinfection and improve the immune response by the efficient recognition of parasite infections and reacting to them. Although research on postbiotics in parasitic diseases is limited, the potential impact of postbiotics on immune function and skin health opens up new perspectives for their future applications [229].

Several advantages can be achieved by the incorporation of postbiotics into topical formulations and skin care products. Postbiotics are stable and, without the need for refrigeration or other elaborate means of storage, can be incorporated into various formulation types: creams, lotions, ointments, and many more. Their stability, therefore, creates suitability for daily use and the fact that they can be applied on the skin in a normal manner. Another merit of postbiotics is that when they are incorporated with other therapeutic medications such as antibiotics or antifungals, they increase their effectiveness and lower the chances that they might develop resistance [255]. Although the prospects presented by postbiotics look very promising, further investigation is still needed in terms of the complete elucidation of the processes in which their mode of action on cutaneous infections takes place and improving the formulation of postbiotics for clinical uses. There is an absolute necessity for clinical trials and investigations to accurately set up the type and amount of postbiotics most useful for treating different skin conditions. It would also be necessary to establish which strain or preparation offers the maximum benefit and to conduct further research on the safety and efficacy of such substances in a variety of distinct populations [256].

Postbiotics and Neurological Infections

Numerous kinds of pathogens may cause neurological diseases. These are inclusive of bacteria, viruses, fungi, and parasites. Because of the need for these microbes to cross the blood-brain barrier, the treatment of severe symptoms, and reducing the risk of long-term neurological damage, such infections-they including meningitis, encephalitis, and neuroinvasive diseases-offer quite substantial challenges. BBB is a selective permeability barrier that often inhibits the effectiveness of conventional therapies; hence, there is a need for new techniques such as postbiotics. Postbiotics have an impact on neurological infections through a variety of methods that could be useful in the treatment of the illnesses. One important step in the process is the immune regulation [258]. The immune system within the central nervous system (CNS) contains a few very specialized cells, including microglia and astrocytes, which are of great significance during the processes taking place in the course of reaction to infections. Postbiotics can modulate the immunological response through the induction of cytokine and chemokine production which is crucial for this process. Such postbiotics have been reported for the enhancement of anti-inflammatory cytokines like IL-10 production with the help of some bacterial strains, which play a crucial role in limiting excessive inflammation and protecting brain tissue [259]. This property of postbiotics, influencing immune cells, will help manage infection and avoid inflammatory damage within the CNS. Besides, the anti-inflammatory effect is one of the major mechanisms attributed to postbiotics. Chronic inflammation may affect the CNS and exacerbate neurological disorders by contributing to neurodegenerative processes. The inflammatory pathways may be inhibited by postbiotics through their action on several transcription factors implicated in the regulation of inflammatory responses, such as NF-kB, which controls the expression of pro-inflammatory genes. These postbiotics might mitigate infections and prevent chronic injuries to brain tissues through the reduction of inflammatory cytokine levels, which could alleviate neuroinflammation [251] (Table 12).

While postbiotics may exert other functional activities, including anti-inflammation modulation, they have the added capability to act antibacterially on microorganisms responsible for diseases of the brain. The postbiotics produced from bacteria like *Lactobacillus* have been shown to possess antibacterial action against pathogens like *E. coli* and *S. aureus* that are implicated in some bacterial infections of the CNS. These can contribute to reducing the pathogenic burden and help resolve the disease condition. Similarly, postbiotics could also possess antiviral properties that may be beneficial for the treatment of viral diseases like herpes simplex encephalitis [259]. Postbiotics contribute to effective infection control by directly interacting with pathogens or enhancing the antimicrobial defenses of host bacteria. Additionally, postbiotics play a role in neuroprotection and healing, particularly in the management of CNS infections. These infections can cause severe damage to neurons, making it crucial to support the brain's repair mechanisms for recovery. Postbiotics likely modulate neurogenesis, the formation of new neurons, and help heal injured neural tissues. Active postbiotics may also stimulate the production of neurotrophic factors, which are essential proteins for neuron survival and development. The potential of postbiotics would reduce the long-term impacts of neurological infections by preserving the integrity of the BBB, thus, on one side, favoring neuronal healing. There are several cases where postbiotics could be employed as a promising treatment strategy for CNS infections [259, 260].

Table 12. Postbiotics and their effects on various infections

Type of Infection	Mechanism of Postbiotic Action	Bioactive Components	Health Benefits	Example Applications
Respiratory Infections	Immune modulation, reduction of inflammation	SCFAs, bacteriocins, antioxidant enzymes	Reduces severity and frequency of infections, improves lung health	Treatment of chronic respiratory diseases (e.g., asthma, bronchitis)
Gastrointestinal Infections	Strengthens gut barrier, prevents pathogen adhesion, reduces inflammation	Exopolysaccharides, SCFAs, peptides	Prevents diarrhea, reduces symptoms of IBD	Therapeutics for IBS, ulcerative colitis
Skin Infections	Antimicrobial effects, anti-inflammatory properties	Teichoic acids, enzymes, EPSs	Reduces acne, eczema, and psoriasis	Topical creams for acne and wound healing
Urinary Tract Infections	Inhibits pathogen colonization, modulates immune response	SCFAs, bacterial lysates	Prevents recurrent infections, strengthens local immunity	Supplements for UTI prevention
Neurological Infections	Reduces systemic inflammation, modulates gut-brain axis	SCFAs, antioxidant enzymes	Improves mental health, reduces inflammation-induced neurological damage	Adjunct therapies for neuroinflammatory conditions
Immunological Infections	Balances the immune system stimulates anti-inflammatory cytokines	Peptidoglycans, lipoteichoic acids	Enhances immunity, reduces autoimmune reactions	Immune-modulating supplements

The postbiotics derived from *Lactobacillus* strains also revealed promising results in these neuroinflammation experimental models, which may change immunological responses, reduce inflammation, and protect against neurodegenerative changes. On the other hand, the postbiotics obtained from *Bifidobacterium* species influence the gut-brain axis; thus, their effect is on the CNS and the gut microbiota. Based on this interaction, the postbiotics obtained from *Bifidobacterium* might have an impact on neuroinflammatory disorders by the action of the CNS and stomach-mediated effect [261]. An antibacterial and anti-inflammatory constituent containing a postbiotic is obtained from a probiotic yeast, *S. boulardii*. Though most of its postbiotics have been studied for their application in the treatment of GI infections, it is not beyond reasonable possibility that these may prove efficacious in the treatment of brain diseases as well. The postbiotics produced by *Saccharomyces boulardii* may therefore serve indirectly in neurological disease management. These postbiotics improve gut health and modulate the immune system at the same time. The potential therapeutic applications of postbiotics extend beyond those described here. Ongoing research continues to uncover new postbiotic compounds and their effects on CNS diseases. To validate these findings, optimize postbiotic formulations, and establish their safety and efficacy across different populations, clinical trials will be necessary [262, 263].

Chapter 10

The Mechanisms of Action of Postbiotics

Abstract

This chapter delves into the mechanisms through which postbiotics exert their biological effects. The interaction between postbiotics and the gut microbiota is explored in depth, highlighting their role in modulating microbial populations and enhancing gut health. The chapter also discusses how postbiotics influence host cell signaling pathways, including the regulation of inflammation, immune responses, and metabolic processes. Additionally, the impact of postbiotics on host gene expression and the modulation of gut-brain communication are examined. The chapter concludes by summarizing the diverse mechanisms through which postbiotics contribute to human health, emphasizing their potential in treating metabolic diseases, gastrointestinal disorders, and neurodegenerative conditions.

Interaction with Gut Microbiota

The gut microbiota represents the grand, complex microbial community colonizing the human gastrointestinal tract, where bacteria, archaea, viruses, and fungi play an important role in human health. This ecosystem is crucial for a wide variety of physiological functions ranging from simple digestion to immunity, or even neurological functions through the gut-brain axis. A balanced gut microbiota is associated with good health, while an imbalance in microbial populations, or a state of dysbiosis, is associated with IBD, obesity, and metabolic syndrome. One of the new therapeutic methods for gut microbiota modulation is the application of postbiotics, namely non-viable microbial metabolites or components derived from probiotics, which confer health benefits to the host [264]. Because postbiotics do not rely on viable microbes for activity, they may be the most promising options because of their stability in safety and efficiency. The postbiotics interact at multiple levels with the intestinal microbiota, influencing not only the composition of microbial populations but also their functionality and providing health benefits. In this respect, examples of such postbiotics are SCFAs, microbial cell wall components, peptides, and EPSs that modulate the gut microbiota and promote the relative growth of beneficial microbes over pathogenic ones. Such a selective modulation of microbial populations is pivotal for the gut ecosystem [265].

One of the major ways gut microbiota and postbiotics interact is in the form of SCFAs, namely, acetate, propionate, and butyrate. These SCFAs result from the fermentation of postbiotic compounds, mainly dietary fibers, by beneficial gut bacteria, including species of *Bifidobacterium* and *Lactobacillus*. SCFAs are an important energy source for colonocytes and generally have anti-inflammatory and immunomodulatory functions. Of these, butyrate is of particular importance for intestinal barrier integrity through the induction of tight junction proteins, preventing entry through the bloodstream by noxious pathogens and toxins. Besides, SCFAs control immune responses through modulation of immune cell activities in gut-associated lymphoid tissue, adding to the overall balance in immune homeostasis [266]. Besides SCFAs, microbial cell wall fragments including peptidoglycans, lipoteichoic acids, and lipopolysaccharides are examples of postbiotics that interact with the host immune system through the engagement of PRRs such as TLRs on the surface of immune cells. Such interactions facilitate the imprinting of the immune response to improve tolerance against beneficial bacteria while defense mechanisms are executed against pathogenic bacteria. All this modulates immune homeostasis, particularly in the gut, which faces constant microbial antigen exposure and thus needs an appropriately tuned immune response [164].

Another important aspect of the interactions between postbiotics and the gut microbiota is the modulation of the intestinal mucus layer. The mucus layer, as known, represents a physical barrier to prevent noxious pathogens from coming into direct contact with the gut epithelium. More importantly, the presence of certain postbiotics, especially those from *Lactobacillus* and *Bifidobacterium* spp., can enhance the expression of the glycoproteins forming the mucus layer- thus improving gut protective functions. Postbiotics maintain gut barrier function by enhancing the production of mucus that acts as a physical barrier, preventing microbial translocation and infection. Besides maintaining gut barrier function, postbiotics exert antimicrobial properties, directly influencing the composition of gut microbiota [267]. For example, bacteriocins are postbiotics and AMPs produced by probiotic bacteria that could impede the growth of pathogenic bacteria by targeting their cell membranes, leading to the lysis of the cell.

Such a kind of selective antimicrobial action favors the growth of helpful bacterial species at the expense of harmful ones, thus favoring a more balanced gut microbiota. Besides this, organic acids, such as lactic acid, synthesized by postbiotics decrease the pH inside the gut and make it unviable for the growth of pathogenic bacteria but supportive of beneficial bacteria [268]. Other aspects of postbiotics include their participation in the cross-talk between gut microbiota and host metabolic processes. By altering the composition of the gut microbiota, postbiotics can modulate the production of bioactive compounds that influence the host's metabolic processes. For example, SCFAs provide energy not only to colonocytes but also help maintain metabolic homeostasis of lipids, glucose, and appetite. Others, such as propionate, among many, were reported to inhibit cholesterol synthesis in the liver, while acetate has been implicated in fat storage and energy expenditure regulation. Metabolic regulation underlines the potential of postbiotics in metabolic disorders such as obesity, type 2 diabetes, and cardiovascular diseases [180].

Intercourse between postbiotics and gut microbiota is not confined to the intestinal cavity but extends further into the systemic immune system and to distant organs through the gut-immune axis and gut-brain axis. For instance, SCFAs have been shown to cross the blood-brain barrier, hence influencing brain functions by modulating neurotransmitter and neurotrophic factor release. Such interaction points to the potential of postbiotics in neurological disorders such as anxiety and depression, as well as neurodegenerative diseases. In this context, their immunomodulatory effects extend beyond the gastrointestinal system and may influence systemic immune responses, helping to alleviate autoimmune diseases and allergic reactions [269]. Postbiotics show promising potential in managing gut microbiota in gastrointestinal disorders such as IBD and IBS. In the case of IBD, a disease characterized by chronic inflammation within the gastrointestinal tract, postbiotics aid in restoring microbial balance and reducing inflammation through anti-inflammatory and immune-regulatory effects. For example, it has been shown that butyrate reduces the levels of pro-inflammatory cytokines and enhances the integrity of the intestinal barrier in IBD patients [270].

The use of postbiotics in IBS might alleviate symptoms like bloating, pain, and altered bowel habits through gut motility modulation and visceral hypersensitivity reduction. Besides, postbiotics may be helpful in the prevention and control of infectious diseases caused by pathogenic bacteria such as *Clostridium difficile*, *Salmonella*, and *E.coli*. Postbiotics, being active substances that modulate gut microbiota composition, can be used to favor the growth of beneficial microbes while limiting or impeding the colonization of pathogenic species, thus reinforcing gut homeostasis and integrity [271]. Thus, the postbiotic SCFAs originating from probiotics inhibited the growth of *C.difficile*, a major cause of antibiotic-associated diarrhea, by acidifying the intestinal environment and increasing the expression of AMPs. Besides their use in the management of gut-related disorders, postbiotics have been shown to influence the gut microbiota in ways that impact metabolic and cardiovascular health in the host. For example, it has been shown that postbiotics may reduce the levels of blood lipids by decreasing the amount of dietary fat and cholesterol absorbed in the intestines, hence reducing the risk for atherosclerosis. Such effects are mediated through the production of SCFAs and other bioactive metabolites with roles in lipid metabolism regulation and inflammation [212].

Recent studies have also pointed out the potential role of postbiotics in the prevention and management of certain types of cancer. The modulation of gut microbiota and reduction of inflammation due to postbiotics may reduce the risk of colorectal cancer associated with dysbiosis and gut chronic inflammation. Besides, antioxidants and anti-inflammatory molecules in some components of postbiotics can inhibit DNA damage and the proliferation of carcinogenic cells. Such features make the interaction of postbiotics with gut microbiota a very promising area of research with far-reaching implications for human health. The modulation of microbial communities and the influence of host physiology by postbiotics open up new frontiers in managing conditions ranging from gastrointestinal disorders to metabolic diseases and even neurological conditions [176]. Hence, due to their stability and safety compared to live probiotics, postbiotics represent a promising alternative for therapeutic intervention, particularly when the use of live microorganisms could be hazardous to populations such as immunocompromised individuals. As research in this area continues to evolve, future studies will likely explore the precise mechanisms through which various postbiotic compounds interact with specific microbial species and how these interactions influence host health. Therefore, personalized postbiotic therapies, tailored to an individual's unique gut microbiota composition, may be the way forward. Additionally, further advancements in manufacturing and delivery methods are crucial to ensuring the maximum therapeutic benefit and effectiveness of these bioactive compounds in clinical settings [272].

Modulation of Host Cell Signaling Pathways

Such manipulation of host-cell signal transduction pathways is dynamic and plays a key role in regulating a wide range of biological processes: immune responses, metabolic control, cell survival, and apoptosis. In turn, host cell signaling pathways represent complex networks of interactions that orchestrate the cell's communication with its immediate surroundings. Impaired regulation may lead from infections and tumors to autoimmune diseases. Of the developing areas of interest, the one that has gained much interest in recent years is how those signaling pathways are influenced by external factors, notably by microbial products-probiotics and postbiotics. Indeed, the interactions between the host cells and microbial components are multifarious in ways that may modulate these pathways at numerous time points, most of which are of paramount importance to human health [273]. Generally, most of these pathways are initiated by the interaction of various signaling molecules, such as hormones, growth factors, or microbial metabolites, which bind to appropriate receptors on the cell surface. These receptors transmit their signals into the cell through a cascade of intracellular events. These cascades often involve the phosphorylation of proteins, activation of kinases, and regulation of gene expression in the nucleus. Among the most famous host cell signaling pathways are the MAPK pathway, NF-κB pathway, PI3K/Akt pathway, and TLR signaling. Each of them plays a very important role in the response of the cell, in modulating the various kinds of external and internal stimuli, including those derived from gut microbiota [274, 275].

The gut microbiota represents a large community of microorganisms, inhabiting the gastrointestinal tract that interacts with host health through the immune system, contributes to metabolic functions, and modulates several host cell signaling pathways. It is also conceivable that the microbes themselves through their secreted products and their metabolic by-products and probiotic strains may affect host cell signaling pathways. The therapeutic potential of gut microbes for the management of inflammation, immune function modulation, and maintenance of intestinal barrier integrity is underpinned by the ability of these organisms to interact with the host signaling network [276]. Among several mechanisms, the interaction between probiotics, microbial-derived metabolites, and host cells involves modulation of the NF-κB signaling pathway. NF-κB is a major regulator of immune responses and inflammation. It regulates the transcription of genes responsible for the synthesis of cytokines, chemokines, and other inflammatory mediators. In unstimulated cells, NF-κB exists as an inactive cytoplasmic complex due to its interaction with a specific inhibitory protein known as IκB. The system is activated, however, after the cell has been exposed to inflammatory signals or microbial components degradation of the inhibitory IκB then allows NF-κB to translocate into the nucleus and generate the pro-inflammatory gene products [277]. Anti-inflammatory properties ascribed to *Lactobacillus* and *Bifidobacterium* species include interference with NF-κB activation. For example, it has been demonstrated that *Lactobacillus rhamnosus* GG prevents IκB degradation, keeping NF-κB in an inactive form, and this decreases transcriptional output of pro-inflammatory cytokines in the intestinal epithelium. Another major signaling pathway targeted by microbial components is the PI3K/Akt pathway. It plays an important role in the pathway responsible for cell survival, metabolism, and growth [275]. Such a pathway is typically activated by the action of growth factors, cytokines, and microbial components. This activation triggers a cascade of events that ultimately promotes cell survival while inhibiting apoptosis. Indeed, it has been demonstrated that probiotics can activate the PI3K/Akt pathway in epithelial cells, promoting cell survival and enhancing barrier function. It is therefore plausible that *Bifidobacterium bifidum* may activate the PI3K/Akt pathway in intestinal epithelial cells, improving intestinal barrier integrity and inhibiting pathogenic invasion [278].

Besides probiotics, postbiotics-metabolic products of probiotics and other intestinal microbiota-also have been shown to influence host cellular signaling. Indeed, postbiotics are diversified and include SCFAs, exopolysaccharides, and bacterial cell wall components. SCFAs are products of gut microbial fermentation of dietary fibers, including acetate, propionate, and butyrate, and exhibit a range of host health-positive effects. Among the most prevalent ways of action through which SCFAs execute their role is by stimulating G-protein-coupled receptors residing on the surface of host cells. These are receptors that take part in transmitting signals from the extracellular environment inside the cell, and the latter could be one of the manners in which SCFAs modulate various signaling pathways implicated in immune responses and metabolic processes [279]. Among SCFAs, butyrate has been considered essential for colonic health since it improves the intestinal barrier and controls the immune response. It has also been shown that butyrate suppresses NF-κB activation, thereby reducing inflammation. Additionally, butyrate activates the peroxisome proliferator-activated receptor gamma (PPARγ) pathway, a key regulator in lipid metabolism and inflammation. Through the activation of PPARγ, butyrate exerts an anti-inflammatory role, contributing to the balance of pro-inflammatory and anti-inflammatory signals in the gut [280].

Another key player in the gut microbiota-host cell interaction is represented by the TLR pathway. TLRs are part of a class of pattern recognition receptors that recognize specific microbe-associated molecular patterns (MAMPs), such as LPS from Gram-negative bacteria and peptidoglycans from Gram-positive bacteria. The recognition of microbial components via TLRs initiates a signaling cascade that leads to the transcription of cytokines and chemokines necessary to initiate an immune response. On the other hand, over-activation of TLR leads to chronic inflammation and tissue damage [133]. Probiotics modulate TLR signaling in a way that represses an overt immune activation, thus leading to a balanced immune response. For example, *L.casei* has been identified to modulate the TLR2 signaling in dendritic cells. This has inhibited the production of pro-inflammatory cytokines while increasing the production of anti-inflammatory cytokines such as IL-10. This crosstalk of probiotics and postbiotics with host cell signaling pathways does not, however, remain limited to the gastrointestinal tract. Indeed, evidence exists that microbial products may influence signal pathways not only in the liver but also within the brain and skin tissues. This is relevant to the gut-brain axis—a bidirectional communication network between the gut and the central nervous system (CNS). Microbial metabolites, including SCFAs and tryptophan metabolites, may influence brain functions and behavior due to their ability to cross the blood-brain barrier. They achieve this by modulating key signaling pathways involved in neurotransmission, neuroinflammation, and neurogenesis [281]. SCFAs, in particular, have been shown to activate G protein-coupled receptors (GPCRs) in the brain, thereby modulating signaling pathways that regulate neuroinflammation and stress responses. This suggests the potential application of both probiotics and postbiotics in treating neurological disorders, including anxiety, depression, and neurodegenerative diseases [282].

Influence on Host Metabolism and Gene Expression

The influence of microbial products, such as probiotics and postbiotics, on host metabolism and gene expression has become very important because it deeply influences human health. The gut microbiota contains trillions of microbes that largely contribute to the sculpting of host physiology by contacting metabolic pathways and influencing gene expression at cellular levels. These microbial communities produce a wide array of metabolites, including SCFAs, vitamins, and amino acids, which may influence host metabolic pathways to affect gene regulation. There is an increasing appreciation that probiotics and postbiotics are indeed powerful regulators of host gene expression not only within the gut but also in peripherally located tissues, thus contributing to a range of physiological outcomes, such as immune homeostasis, metabolic balance, and the prevention of illness [283]. The gut microbiota's ability to process complex dietary compounds indigestible by the human host is central to microbial influence on host metabolism. For instance, dietary fibers are metabolized into SCFAs such as acetate, propionate, and butyrate by gut bacteria. These SCFAs get absorbed through the host cells, where they act further as energy sources and signaling molecules. Among these products, butyrate is particularly important because of its key role in the regulation of gene expression. Butyrate exerts this effect because it is an inhibitor of histone deacetylases. Inhibiting histone deacetylases, butyrate promotes acetylation of histones-a process that relaxes the structure of the chromatin and allows for the transcription of particular genes. In this regard, butyrate may modulate genes implicated in the regulation of inflammation, cell proliferation, and programmed cell death, thus influencing processes such as immune regulation and tissue repair [284]. Besides the action of butyrate on epigenetic regulation, the other SCFAs-acetate and propionate- exert an effect on metabolic pathways because of their capability to activate particular host cell receptors. One example includes G-protein-coupled receptor 43, which is activated by propionate and also acetate. This activation of GPR43 is followed by intracellular cascades that result in influences on glucose and lipid metabolisms. For instance, it has been demonstrated that the activation of GPR43 reduces insulin resistance and increases lipid oxidation in the adipose tissue, thus having a protective function against metabolic disorders, including obesity and type 2 diabetes. This possibility of modulation by SCFAs of these metabolic pathways points out the complex relationship between gut microbiota and host metabolism and might have a therapeutic perspective in metabolic disorders management [285].

Another main area of interaction between microbial products and host metabolic function involves the synthesis and production of bile acids and their derivatives. Bile acids, which are synthesized in the liver by conversion of cholesterol, are secreted into the intestine, where they exert an important function in food fat digestion and absorption. However, gut bacteria can metabolize primary bile acids into secondary ones that may control the host gene expression involved in the regulation of lipid metabolism, glucose homeostasis, and energy expenditure upon activation of nuclear receptors such as farnesoid X receptor (FXR) and Takeda G-protein-coupled receptor 5 (TGR5) [286]. For instance, activation of FXR by bile acids has been shown to inhibit lipogenesis and stimulate fatty acid oxidation, thus playing a protective role against non-alcoholic fatty liver disease (NAFLD) and atherosclerosis. The modification of bile acids by gut bacteria, along with the subsequent regulation of host gene expression, is a key aspect of microbial influence on host metabolism. Probiotics, which are viable microorganisms that confer health benefits when administered in adequate amounts, have also been found to play important roles in modulating host metabolism and gene expression. Species from *Lactobacillus* and *Bifidobacterium* have been found to influence the expression of genes related to lipid metabolism, inflammation, and immune responses [287]. One way they do this is by modulating TLR signaling. TLRs represent a family of PRRs recognizing MAMPs, thereby inducing intracellular signaling cascades that activate various transcription factors, including NF-κB. Probiotics modulate TLR signaling to dampen the inflammatory response and induce anti-inflammatory gene expression. For example, *L.rhamnosus* GG was found to downregulate the expression of pro-inflammatory genes in intestinal epithelial cells via the inhibition of NF-κB activation and thus to be involved in the maintenance of intestinal homeostasis [288].

Probiotics also affect the host metabolism through the modulation of activities of enzymes connected with both the synthesis and degradation of lipids. For example, *B.longum* enhances the expression of the peroxisome proliferator-activated receptor alpha gene in the liver, which is involved in fatty acid oxidation and accelerates the degradation of fatty acids while impeding fat accumulation in the liver. These are indications that probiotics may have therapeutic value in the management of metabolic disorders such as NAFLD. It also has been shown that *L.plantarum* modulates the expression of genes related to cholesterol metabolism and lowers the level of cholesterol in the blood. This property of the probiotics, to affect lipid metabolism, is an important aspect of the prevention of cardiovascular diseases. Besides the gut, metabolites produced by microbes can affect gene expression and metabolic pathways of other organs via the gut-liver and gut-brain axes [289]. The gut-liver axis refers to the bidirectional communication between the gut microbiota and the liver, which is mediated by microbial metabolites, including SCFAs and BA. As already mentioned, such metabolites can modulate gene expression in the liver by their action on nuclear receptors FXR and PPARα. In addition to their role in lipid metabolism, microbial metabolites may also modulate liver inflammation and fibrosis, which is an important aspect of the disease process in both NAFLD and cirrhosis. The gut-brain axis communicates with both the gut microbiota and the CNS through microbial metabolites, immune signaling, and the vagus nerve. SCFAs and tryptophan metabolites could affect gene expression in the brain through influence on neuroinflammation, neurogenesis, and neurotransmission by crossing the blood-brain barrier. All of these might hint at a possible therapeutic intervention in neurological disorders, including depression and anxiety or even neurodegenerative diseases [290, 291].

Nonviable microbial products, metabolic by-products, or what has been referred to recently as postbiotics, could also influence host metabolism and gene expression. Postbiotics represent a diverse group of bioactive molecules, including SCFAs, exopolysaccharides, and bacterial cell wall components that can modulate metabolic and immune responses. As previously discussed, SCFAs are key postbiotics that directly modulate host gene expression through histone deacetylase (HDAC) inhibition and GPCR activation. EPSs are polysaccharides secreted by bacteria and, similarly, have been shown to influence host gene expression. For instance, EPSs produced by *L.rhamnosus* can induce signaling pathways that are part of immune regulation and promote the secretion of anti-inflammatory cytokines such as IL-10 [111, 292]. This sort of immunomodulatory effect imparted by the postbiotics may have some therapeutic advantages in inflammatory diseases and autoimmune disorders. Besides immune regulation, postbiotics can also impact host metabolic pathways by modulating the expression of genes involved with energy homeostasis. For instance, peptidoglycan and lipoteichoic acid of bacterial cell walls have been known to activate TLRs along with other pattern recognition receptors on the host cells, which may initiate downstream signaling pathways that ultimately regulate energy metabolism. These interactions can influence the expression of genes involved in glucose uptake, insulin sensitivity, and lipid metabolism, thereby contributing to the maintenance of metabolic homeostasis. The role of postbiotics in modulating gene expression highlights their potential therapeutic applications in metabolic disorders such as obesity, type 2 diabetes, and cardiovascular diseases [293].

Table 13. Mechanisms of action of postbiotics

Mechanism	Description	Bioactive Components	Health Effects	Example Applications
Immune Modulation	Balances pro- and anti-inflammatory cytokines, activates immune cells	Peptidoglycans, SCFAs, teichoic acids	Reduces chronic inflammation, strengthens immunity	Treatment for autoimmune and inflammatory diseases
Gut Barrier Enhancement	Promotes production of tight junction proteins, increases mucin secretion	SCFAs, exopolysaccharides, peptides	Prevents leaky gut, reduces pathogen translocation	Therapies for IBD, IBS, and gastrointestinal health
Antimicrobial Activity	Inhibits pathogen growth and adhesion, disrupts microbial membranes	Bacteriocins, lipoteichoic acids, enzymes	Prevents infections, reduces antibiotic dependence	Antibiotic alternatives, infection prevention
Oxidative Stress Reduction	Neutralizes ROS supports antioxidant defense systems	Antioxidant enzymes (SOD, CAT, GPx)	Protects against cellular damage, reduces aging effects	Skincare products, cardiovascular health
Metabolic Regulation	Modulates glucose and lipid metabolism and supports SCFA production	SCFAs (butyrate, propionate, acetate)	Improves insulin sensitivity, reduces obesity	Supplements for metabolic disorders
Microbiota Modulation	Enhances the growth of beneficial bacteria, inhibits harmful pathogens	SCFAs, exopolysaccharides	Restores microbiota balance, improves digestion	Functional foods, probiotics, synbiotics
Neuroprotective Effects	Influences gut-brain axis, reduces systemic and neural inflammation	SCFAs, peptides	Supports mental health, reduces neurodegenerative risks	Adjunct treatments for anxiety, depression

It would be an over-simplification to assume that such an influence of microbial products on host gene expression is restricted to metabolic and immune responses. Microbes and their metabolites can also modulate genes associated with epithelial barrier function, tissue repair, and cell proliferation. The intestinal epithelium is a crucial barrier between the host and the external environment. Loss of its integrity can allow the translocation of infectious agents and toxic substances from the gut lumen into the bloodstream. Microbial products, such as butyrate, enhance the expression of tight junction proteins, which are essential for maintaining the integrity of the intestinal barrier. Because microbial products promote the expression of those proteins, barrier dysfunction is evaded, and the risk of diseases such as IBD and colorectal cancer is reduced [294]. Other genes whose expressions are modulated by probiotics and postbiotics are those involved in tissue repair and cell proliferation. Thus, *L. acidophilus* enhanced epidermal growth factor expression and its receptor on the intestinal epithelial cells and consequently increased cell proliferation and tissue repair. Thus, this suggests that, in the future, probiotics may be used as therapeutic agents for healing injured tissues, particularly in the gastrointestinal tract. Similarly, SCFAs such as butyrate have been shown to suppress pro-apoptotic gene expression while inducing anti-apoptotic genes in the intestinal epithelium, thereby promoting cell survival and contributing to tissue homeostasis [295] (Table 13).

Conclusion

The functionality of postbiotics in a variety of therapeutic scenarios demonstrates that these non-viable microbial compounds or metabolites have significant medicinal and clinical potential. Most research on postbiotics explores their diverse applications, including effects on gastrointestinal, urinary, respiratory, and dermal infections, as well as neurological disorders. The following review highlights the complexity of postbiotics and their potential to uncover innovative solutions for addressing multifaceted health issues. As stable and non-viable metabolic products of microbial fermentation or cellular components, postbiotics offer several advantages over active probiotics. Their stability and safety make them suitable for numerous applications, including cases where the survival of living microbes is not possible. Postbiotics exhibit a wide range of bioactivities, including antibacterial, anti-inflammatory, immune-modulating, and neuroprotective effects, which support their use as therapeutic agents in various areas of medicine.

Detailed mechanisms of action, such as immune regulation, anti-inflammatory effects, antibacterial properties, and facilitation of tissue repair, highlight the critical roles that postbiotics play in combating infections and restoring health across various organ systems. For example, in gastrointestinal infections, postbiotics have the potential to enhance gut barrier integrity and modulate gut microbiota, thereby contributing to overall health and infection control. Similarly, their involvement in urinary and respiratory infections, as well as dermatological disorders, demonstrates their ability to actively combat pathogens and enhance both systemic and localized immune responses. In neurological infections, postbiotics offer a novel approach to addressing complex disorders affecting the central and peripheral nervous systems. Their potential for modulating neuroinflammation, along with enhancing neuroprotection and reparative processes, opens up new possibilities for managing severe, often intractable diseases.

Postbiotics could, therefore, represent a significant addition to therapeutic strategies in neurological diseases by orchestrating immunomodulatory effects while also promoting brain health. The following book provides a comprehensive review of postbiotics and their potential to revolutionize various aspects of medical practice. These examples and data are presented to demonstrate how postbiotics can help address existing challenges in infection control and treatment strategies. Further research is necessary to fully establish their efficacy and safety, as well as to refine their formulation and extend their applications through studies and clinical trials. Postbiotics represent a promising area of medical research. Their diverse mechanisms of action and unique characteristics make them highly promising for health improvements across a wide range of diseases. Clinical applications and extensive research into the benefits of postbiotics will hopefully lead to new therapeutic and preventive options, ultimately improving patient outcomes and overall quality of life.

References

[1] Sabahi S, Homayouni Rad A, Aghebati-Maleki L, Sangtarash N, Ozma MA, Karimi A, et al. Postbiotics as the new frontier in food and pharmaceutical research. *Critical reviews in food science and nutrition.* 2023;63(26):8375-402.

[2] Patra JK, Das G, Paramithiotis S, Shin H-S. Kimchi and other widely consumed traditional fermented foods of Korea: a review. *Frontiers in microbiology.* 2016;7:1493.

[3] Nezhadi J, Rezaee MA, Ozma MA, Ganbarov K, Kafil HS. Gut Microbiota Exchange in Domestic Animals and Rural-urban People Axis. *Current Pharmaceutical Biotechnology.* 2024.

[4] Wang X, Zhang P, Zhang X. Probiotics regulate gut microbiota: an effective method to improve immunity. *Molecules.* 2021;26(19):6076.

[5] Yakout HM, Eckhardt E. Gastrointestinal tract barrier efficiency: function and threats. *Gut Microbiota, Immunity, and Health in Production Animals*: Springer; 2022. p. 13-32.

[6] Mirzaei R, Kavyani B, Nabizadeh E, Kadkhoda H, Ozma MA, Abdi M. Microbiota metabolites in the female reproductive system: Focused on the short-chain fatty acids. *Heliyon.* 2023.

[7] Liu Y, Tran DQ, Rhoads JM. Probiotics in disease prevention and treatment. *The Journal of Clinical Pharmacology.* 2018;58:S164-S79.

[8] Ray RC, Paramithiotis S, Thekkangil A, Nethravathy V, Rai AK, Martin JGP. Food Fermentation and Its Relevance in the Human History. *Trending Topics on Fermented Foods:* Springer; 2024. p. 1-57.

[9] Tamang JP, Cotter PD, Endo A, Han NS, Kort R, Liu SQ, et al. Fermented foods in a global age: East meets West. *Comprehensive Reviews in Food Science and Food Safety.* 2020;19(1):184-217.

[10] Underhill DM, Gordon S, Imhof BA, Núñez G, Bousso P. Élie Metchnikoff (1845–1916): celebrating 100 years of cellular immunology and beyond. *Nature Reviews Immunology.* 2016;16(10):651-6.

[11] Saulnier DM, Kolida S, Gibson GR. Microbiology of the human intestinal tract and approaches for its dietary modulation. *Current Pharmaceutical Design.* 2009;15(13):1403-14.

[12] Bhat A. *Bacterial production of poly-γ-glutamic acid and evaluation of its effect on the viability of probiotic microorganisms.* 2012.

[13] Ozma MA, Moaddab SR, Hosseini H, Khodadadi E, Ghotaslou R, Asgharzadeh M, et al. A critical review of novel antibiotic resistance prevention approaches

with a focus on postbiotics. *Critical Reviews in Food Science and Nutrition.* 2023:1-19.

[14] Arora M, Baldi A. Regulatory categories of probiotics across the globe: a review representing existing and recommended categorization. *Indian journal of medical microbiology.* 2015;33:S2-S10.

[15] Papadimitriou K, Zoumpopoulou G, Foligné B, Alexandraki V, Kazou M, Pot B, Tsakalidou E. Discovering probiotic microorganisms: in vitro, in vivo, genetic and omics approaches. *Frontiers in microbiology.* 2015;6:58.

[16] Ozma MA, Abbasi A, Sabahi S. Characterization of postbiotics derived from Lactobacillus paracasei ATCC 55544 and its application in Malva sylvestris seed mucilage edible coating to the improvement of the microbiological, and sensory properties of lamb meat during storage. *Biointerface Res Appl Chem.* 2022;13.

[17] Desai A. *Strain identification, viability and probiotics properties of Lactobacillus casei:* Victoria University; 2008.

[18] Kailasapathy K, Chin J. Survival and therapeutic potential of probiotic organisms with reference to Lactobacillus acidophilus and Bifidobacterium spp. *Immunology and cell biology.* 2000;78(1):80-8.

[19] McFarland LV. Systematic review and meta-analysis of Saccharomyces boulardii in adult patients. *World journal of gastroenterology: WJG.* 2010;16(18):2202.

[20] Huang Y-Y, Lu Y-H, Liu X-T, Wu W-T, Li W-Q, Lai S-Q, et al. Metabolic properties, functional characteristics, and practical application of Streptococcus thermophilus. *Food Reviews International.* 2024;40(2):792-813.

[21] Bravo Santano N, Juncker Boll E, Catrine Capern L, Cieplak TM, Keleszade E, Letek M, Costabile A. Comparative evaluation of the antimicrobial and mucus induction properties of selected Bacillus strains against enterotoxigenic Escherichia coli. *Antibiotics.* 2020;9(12):849.

[22] Koenraad VH, Vandamme P, Vervaecke S, Anita VL. Maldi-Tof MS of microbial mixtures: impressions of its usability for culture-independent analyses of microbial diversity in food ecosystems. *The Challenge of Complexity MD2015.* 2015:162.

[23] Hatoum R, Labrie S, Fliss I. Antimicrobial and probiotic properties of yeasts: from fundamental to novel applications. *Frontiers in microbiology.* 2012;3:421.

[24] Derrien M, Belzer C, de Vos WM. Akkermansia muciniphila and its role in regulating host functions. *Microbial pathogenesis.* 2017;106:171-81.

[25] Abbasi A, Bazzaz S, Da Cruz AG, Khorshidian N, Saadat YR, Sabahi S, et al. A Critical Review on Akkermansia Muciniphila: Functional Mechanisms, Technological Challenges, and Safety Issues. *Probiotics and Antimicrobial Proteins.* 2023:1-23.

[26] Ghotaslou R, Nabizadeh E, Memar MY, Law WMH, Ozma MA, Abdi M, et al. The metabolic, protective, and immune functions of Akkermansia muciniphila. *Microbiological Research.* 2023;266:127245.

[27] 박영태. Physiological activity of butyrate-producing gut bacteria: 서울대학교 대학원; 2019.

[28] Cassir N, Benamar S, La Scola B. Clostridium butyricum: from beneficial to a new emerging pathogen. *Clinical Microbiology and Infection.* 2016;22(1):37-45.

[29] Sonnenborn U. Escherichia coli strain Nissle 1917—from bench to bedside and back: history of a special Escherichia coli strain with probiotic properties. *FEMS microbiology letters.* 2016;363(19):fnw212.

[30] Elshaghabee FM, Rokana N, Gulhane RD, Sharma C, Panwar H. Bacillus as potential probiotics: status, concerns, and future perspectives. *Frontiers in microbiology.* 2017;8:1490.

[31] Bentzon-Tilia M, Gram L. Biotechnological applications of the Roseobacter clade. *Bioprospecting: Success, potential and constraints.* 2017:137-66.

[32] Verma P, Dutt R, Anwar S. Effect of probiotic Lactobacillus helveticus on various health disorders. *Current Traditional Medicine.* 2023;9(4):105-13.

[33] Bienenstock J, Gibson G, Klaenhammer TR, Walker WA, Neish AS. New insights into probiotic mechanisms: a harvest from functional and metagenomic studies. *Gut microbes.* 2013;4(2):94-100.

[34] Khomeiri M, Taheri S, Nasrollahzadeh A. Non-LAB Bacterial Probiotic: Next-Generation Probiotic, Bacillus Spp., Clostridium butyricum. *Handbook of Food Bioactive Ingredients: Properties and Applications:* Springer; 2023. p. 1-28.

[35] Ozma MA, Abbasi A, Ahangarzadeh Rezaee M, Hosseini H, Hosseinzadeh N, Sabahi S, et al. A critical review on the nutritional and medicinal profiles of garlic's (Allium sativum L.) bioactive compounds. *Food Reviews International.* 2023;39(9):6324-61.

[36] Gibson GR, Probert HM, Van Loo J, Rastall RA, Roberfroid MB. Dietary modulation of the human colonic microbiota: updating the concept of prebiotics. *Nutrition research reviews.* 2004;17(2):259-75.

[37] Guarino MPL, Altomare A, Emerenziani S, Di Rosa C, Ribolsi M, Balestrieri P, et al. Mechanisms of action of prebiotics and their effects on gastro-intestinal disorders in adults. *Nutrients.* 2020;12(4):1037.

[38] Rajagopalan G, Krishnan C. Functional oligosaccharides: production and action. *Next generation biomanufacturing technologies:* ACS Publications; 2019. p. 155-80.

[39] Liburdi K, Esti M. Galacto-oligosaccharide (GOS) synthesis during enzymatic lactose-free Milk production: state of the art and emerging opportunities. *Beverages.* 2022;8(2):21.

[40] Mudannayake DC, Jayasena DD, Wimalasiri KM, Ranadheera CS, Ajlouni S. Inulin fructans–food applications and alternative plant sources: a review. *International Journal of Food Science & Technology.* 2022;57(9):5764-80.

[41] Wouters R. Inulin. Food stabilisers, thickeners and gelling agents. 2009:180-97.

[42] Topping DL, Clifton PM. Short-chain fatty acids and human colonic function: roles of resistant starch and nonstarch polysaccharides. *Physiological reviews.* 2001;81(3):1031-64.

[43] Pérez-Escalante E, Alatorre-Santamaría S, Castañeda-Ovando A, Salazar-Pereda V, Bautista-Ávila M, Cruz-Guerrero AE, et al. Human milk oligosaccharides as bioactive compounds in infant formula: recent advances and trends in synthetic methods. *Critical Reviews in Food Science and Nutrition.* 2022;62(1):181-214.

[44] Wang J, Chen C, Yu Z, He Y, Yong Q, Newburg DS. Relative fermentation of oligosaccharides from human milk and plants by gut microbes. *European Food Research and Technology.* 2017;243:133-46.

[45] Sorndech W, Nakorn KN, Tongta S, Blennow A. Isomalto-oligosaccharides: Recent insights in production technology and their use for food and medical applications. *Lwt.* 2018;95:135-42.

[46] Thammarutwasik P, Hongpattarakere T, Chantachum S, Kijroongrojana K, Itharat A, Reanmongkol W, et al. Prebiotics-A Review. *Songklanakarin Journal of Science & Technology.* 2009;31(4).

[47] Perović J, Šaponjac VT, Kojić J, Krulj J, Moreno DA, García-Viguera C, et al. Chicory (Cichorium intybus L.) as a food ingredient–Nutritional composition, bioactivity, safety, and health claims: A review. *Food chemistry.* 2021;336:127676.

[48] Khalid W, Arshad MS, Jabeen A, Muhammad Anjum F, Qaisrani TB, Suleria HAR. Fiber-enriched botanicals: A therapeutic tool against certain metabolic ailments. *Food Science & Nutrition.* 2022;10(10):3203-18.

[49] Daou C, Zhang H. Oat beta-glucan: its role in health promotion and prevention of diseases. *Comprehensive reviews in food science and food safety.* 2012;11(4):355-65.

[50] Annor GA, Ma Z, Boye JI. Crops–legumes. *Food processing: principles and applications.* 2014:305-37.

[51] Keskin SO, Ali TM, Ahmed J, Shaikh M, Siddiq M, Uebersax MA. Physico-chemical and functional properties of legume protein, starch, and dietary fiber—A review. *Legume Science.* 2022;4(1):e117.

[52] Sanderson H. Roots and tubers. *The cultural history of plants: Routledge*; 2012. p. 66-81.

[53] Kalinik E. *Be Good to Your Gut: The ultimate guide to gut health-with 80 delicious recipes to feed your body and mind:* Hachette UK; 2017.

[54] Praznik W, Loeppert R, Viernstein H, Haslberger AG, Unger FM. Dietary fiber and prebiotics. *Polysaccharides: Bioactivity and Biotechnology Cham:* Springer International Publishing. 2015:891-925.

[55] Verma R, Saxena G. *The Gut Micro-Biota and Health Benefits of Probiotics, Prebiotics & Synbiotics.*

[56] Gomte SS, Rout B, Agnihotri TG, Peddinti V, Jain A. Future Perspective and Safety Issues of Synbiotics in Different Diseases. *Synbiotics in Human Health: Biology to Drug Delivery:* Springer; 2024. p. 281-307.

[57] Mehjabin S, Akanda MKM, Hasan AN, Parvez GM. Synbiotics: Present Status and Future Prospectives to Control Metabolic Disorders. *Synbiotics in Metabolic Disorders:* CRC Press. p. 245-56.

[58] Abbasi A, Bazzaz S, A. Ibrahim S, Hekmatdoost A, Hosseini H, Sabahi S, et al. A critical review on the gluten-induced enteropathy/celiac disease: gluten-targeted dietary and non-dietary therapeutic approaches. *Food Reviews International.* 2024;40(3):883-923.

[59] Ngoc APT, Zahoor A, Kim DG, Yang SH. Using Synbiotics as a Therapy to Protect Mental Health in Alzheimer's Disease. *Journal of Microbiology and Biotechnology.* 2024;34(9):1739.

[60] Simpson P. *Good Bacteria for Healthy Skin: Nurture Your Skin Microbiome with Pre-and Probiotics for Clear and Luminous Skin*: Simon and Schuster; 2019.

[61] Żółkiewicz J, Marzec A, Ruszczyński M, Feleszko W. Postbiotics—a step beyond pre-and probiotics. *Nutrients.* 2020;12(8):2189.

[62] Karani NG, Uzzal KK, Omoikhoje ID. *Probiotics as Promising Therapeutics: A Review of Literature.*

[63] Yeşilyurt N, Yılmaz B, Ağagündüz D, Capasso R. Involvement of probiotics and postbiotics in the immune system modulation. *Biologics.* 2021;1(2):89-110.

[64] de Almada CN, Almada CN, Martinez RC, Sant'Ana AS. Paraprobiotics: Evidences on their ability to modify biological responses, inactivation methods and perspectives on their application in foods. *Trends in food science & technology.* 2016;58:96-114.

[65] Kumar H, Schütz F, Bhardwaj K, Sharma R, Nepovimova E, Dhanjal DS, et al. Recent advances in the concept of paraprobiotics: Nutraceutical/functional properties for promoting children health. *Critical Reviews in Food Science and Nutrition.* 2023;63(19):3943-58.

[66] Panitsidis I, Barbe F, Chevaux E, Giannenas I, Demey V. Probiotics, prebiotics, paraprobiotics, postbiotics. *Sustainable use of feed additives in livestock: Novel ways for animal production:* Springer; 2023. p. 173-227.

[67] Dinan TG, Stanton C, Cryan JF. Psychobiotics: a novel class of psychotropic. *Biol Psychiatry.* 2013;74(10):720-6.

[68] Meher AK, Acharya B, Sahu PK. Probiotics: Bridging the interplay of a healthy gut and psychoneurological well-being. *Food Bioengineering.* 2024;3(1):126-47.

[69] Bermúdez-Humarán LG, Salinas E, Ortiz GG, Ramirez-Jirano LJ, Morales JA, Bitzer-Quintero OK. From probiotics to psychobiotics: live beneficial bacteria which act on the brain-gut axis. *Nutrients.* 2019;11(4):890.

[70] Dziedzic A, Maciak K, Bliźniewska-Kowalska K, Gałecka M, Kobierecka W, Saluk J. The Power of Psychobiotics in Depression: A Modern Approach through the Microbiota–Gut–Brain Axis: A Literature Review. *Nutrients.* 2024;16(7):1054.

[71] Trzeciak P, Herbet M. Role of the intestinal microbiome, intestinal barrier and psychobiotics in depression. *Nutrients.* 2021;13(3):927.

[72] Ross K. Psychobiotics: Are they the future intervention for managing depression and anxiety? A literature review. *Explore.* 2023;19(5):669-80.

[73] Dehghani F, Abdollahi S, Shidfar F, Clark CC, Soltani S. Probiotics supplementation and brain-derived neurotrophic factor (BDNF): A systematic review and meta-analysis of randomized controlled trials. *Nutritional neuroscience.* 2023;26(10):942-52.

[74] Dhyani P, Goyal C, Dhull SB, Chauhan AK, Singh Saharan B, Harshita, et al. Psychobiotics for mitigation of neuro-degenerative diseases: Recent advancements. *Molecular nutrition & food research.* 2024;68(13):2300461.

[75] Tripathi A, Pandey VK, Tiwari V, Mishra R, Dash KK, Harsányi E, et al. Exploring the Fermentation-Driven Functionalities of Lactobacillaceae-Originated Probiotics in Preventive Measures of Alzheimer's Disease: A Review. *Fermentation.* 2023;9(8):762.

[76] Bhatt B, Patel K, Lee CN, Moochhala S. *The Microbial Blueprint: The Impact of Your Gut on Your Well-being:* Partridge Publishing Singapore; 2024.

[77] Villena J, Kitazawa H. immunobiotics—interactions of Beneficial Microbes with the immune System. *Frontiers Media SA;* 2017. p. 1580.

[78] Salva S, Kolling Y, Ivir M, Gutiérrez F, Alvarez S. The role of immunobiotics and postbiotics in the recovery of immune cell populations from respiratory mucosa of malnourished hosts: effect on the resistance against respiratory infections. *Frontiers in Nutrition.* 2021;8:704868.

[79] Khaskheli AA, Khaskheli MI, Khaskheli AJ, Khaskheli AA. A review on the influence of dietary immunobiotics on the performance, intestinal morphology and immune-related gene expression in post-hatched broiler chicks. *Aceh Journal of Animal Science.* 2020;5(1):57-67.

[80] Shigemori S, Shimosato T. Applications of genetically modified immunobiotics with high immunoregulatory capacity for treatment of inflammatory bowel diseases. *Frontiers in immunology*. 2017;8:22.

[81] Mal S, Das TK, Pradhan S, Ghosh K. Probiotics as a Therapeutic Approach for Non-infectious Gastric Ulcer Management: a Comprehensive Review. *Probiotics and Antimicrobial Proteins.* 2024:1-26.

[82] Villena J, Salva S, Barbieri N, Alvarez S. Immunobiotics for the prevention of bacterial and viral respiratory infections. *Probiotics: Immunobiotics and Immunogenics:* Science Publishers, CRC Press, Taylor & Francis Group company. 2013:128-68.

[83] Raheem A, Liang L, Zhang G, Cui S. Modulatory effects of probiotics during pathogenic infections with emphasis on immune regulation. *Frontiers in immunology*. 2021;12:616713.

[84] Tarsillo B, Priefer R. Proteobiotics as a new antimicrobial therapy. *Microbial pathogenesis.* 2020;142:104093.

[85] TENEA GN. Postbiotics: a solution to protect tropical fruits towards postharvest adulteration. *AgroLife Scientific Journal.* 2021;10(2).

[86] Pires L, González-Paramás AM, Heleno SA, Calhelha RC. Exploring therapeutic advances: a comprehensive review of intestinal microbiota modulators. *Antibiotics.* 2024;13(8):720.

[87] Canibe N, Højberg O, Kongsted H, Vodolazska D, Lauridsen C, Nielsen TS, Schönherz AA. Review on preventive measures to reduce post-weaning diarrhoea in piglets. *Animals.* 2022;12(19):2585.

[88] Bourebaba Y, Marycz K, Mularczyk M, Bourebaba L. Postbiotics as potential new therapeutic agents for metabolic disorders management. *Biomedicine & Pharmacotherapy*. 2022;153:113138.

[89] Wilson RM. *Investigating the Antibacterial and Immunomodulatory Properties of Lactobacillus acidophilus Postbiotics*. 2023.

[90] Gurunathan S, Thangaraj P, Kim J-H. Postbiotics: functional food materials and therapeutic agents for cancer, diabetes, and inflammatory diseases. *Foods.* 2023;13(1):89.

[91] Warda AK, Clooney AG, Ryan F, de Almeida Bettio PH, Di Benedetto G, Ross RP, Hill C. A postbiotic consisting of heat-treated lactobacilli has a bifidogenic effect in pure culture and in human fermented fecal communities. *Applied and environmental microbiology.* 2021;87(8):e02459-20.

[92] Moradi M, Molaei R, Guimarães JT. A review on preparation and chemical analysis of postbiotics from lactic acid bacteria. *Enzyme and Microbial Technology.* 2021;143:109722.

[93] Dahiya R, Khan S, Kumar S. A Review on Probiotics and Their Role in the Management of Cancer. *Current Probiotics.* 2024;1(1):e120124225596.

[94] De Silva A, Bloom SR. Gut hormones and appetite control: a focus on PYY and GLP-1 as therapeutic targets in obesity. *Gut and liver.* 2012;6(1):10.

[95] Wu W, Chen Z, Han J, Qian L, Wang W, Lei J, Wang H. Endocrine, genetic, and microbiome nexus of obesity and potential role of postbiotics: a narrative review. *Eating and Weight Disorders-Studies on Anorexia, Bulimia and Obesity.* 2023;28(1):84.

[96] Mahdavi S, Ozma MA, Azadi A, Sadeghi J, Baghi HB, Oskouee MA. Interaction of the viral infectious agents in the development and exacerbation of the multiple sclerosis. *Le Infezioni in Medicina.* 2023;31(4):476.

[97] Stengler M. *The Holistic Guide to Gut Health: Discover the Truth About Leaky Gut, Balancing Your Microbiome, and Restoring Whole-Body Health*: Hay House, Inc; 2024.

[98] Fan Y, Gu R, Zhang R, Wang M, Xu H, Wang M, Long C. Protective effects of extracts from Acer truncatum leaves on SLS-induced HaCaT cells. *Frontiers in Pharmacology.* 2023;14:1068849.

[99] Chen Z, Yang Y, Cui X, Chai L, Liu H, Pan Y, et al. Process, advances, and perspectives of graphene oxide-SELEX for the development of aptamer molecular probes: A comprehensive review. *Analytica Chimica Acta.* 2024:343004.

[100] Chatzopoulou S, Eriksson NL, Eriksson D. Improving risk assessment in the European food safety authority: lessons from the European Medicines Agency. *Frontiers in Plant Science.* 2020;11:349.

[101] Abdilla N, Tormo M, Fabia M, Chaves F, Saez G, Redon J. Impact of the components of metabolic syndrome on oxidative stress and enzymatic antioxidant activity in essential hypertension. *Journal of Human Hypertension.* 2007;21(1):68-75.

[102] Sahoo BM, Banik BK, Borah P, Jain A. Reactive oxygen species (ROS): key components in cancer therapies. *Anti-Cancer Agents in Medicinal Chemistry (Formerly Current Medicinal Chemistry-Anti-Cancer Agents).* 2022;22(2):215-22.

[103] Hasanuzzaman M, Bhuyan MB, Zulfiqar F, Raza A, Mohsin SM, Mahmud JA, et al. Reactive oxygen species and antioxidant defense in plants under abiotic stress:

Revisiting the crucial role of a universal defense regulator. *Antioxidants.* 2020;9(8):681.

[104] Razack SA, Velayutham V, Thangavelu V. Medium optimization for the production of exopolysaccharide by Bacillus subtilis using synthetic sources and agro wastes. *Turkish Journal of Biology.* 2013;37(3):280-8.

[105] Juan CA, Pérez de la Lastra JM, Plou FJ, Pérez-Lebeña E. The chemistry of reactive oxygen species (ROS) revisited: outlining their role in biological macromolecules (DNA, lipids and proteins) and induced pathologies. *International journal of molecular sciences.* 2021;22(9):4642.

[106] Wang Y, Wu Y, Wang Y, Xu H, Mei X, Yu D, et al. Antioxidant properties of probiotic bacteria. *Nutrients.* 2017;9(5):521.

[107] Suliman HB, Piantadosi CA. Mitochondrial quality control as a therapeutic target. *Pharmacological reviews*. 2016;68(1):20-48.

[108] Bartsch H, Nair J. Chronic inflammation and oxidative stress in the genesis and perpetuation of cancer: role of lipid peroxidation, DNA damage, and repair. *Langenbeck's Archives of Surgery.* 2006;391:499-510.

[109] Shirkhan F, Safaei F, Mirdamadi S, Zandi M. The Role of Probiotics in Skin Care: Advances, Challenges, and Future Needs. *Probiotics and Antimicrobial Proteins*. 2024:1-18.

[110] Tai S. Comparing approaches towards governing scientific advisory bodies on food safety in the United States and the European Union. *Wis L Rev.* 2010:627.

[111] Prajapati N, Patel J, Singh S, Yadav VK, Joshi C, Patani A, et al. Postbiotic production: harnessing the power of microbial metabolites for health applications. *Frontiers in Microbiology.* 2023;14:1306192.

[112] Kupnik K, Primožič M, Vasić K, Knez Ž, Leitgeb M. A comprehensive study of the antibacterial activity of bioactive juice and extracts from pomegranate (Punica granatum L.) peels and seeds. *Plants.* 2021;10(8):1554.

[113] Dama A, Shpati K, Daliu P, Dumur S, Gorica E, Santini A. Targeting metabolic diseases: the role of nutraceuticals in modulating oxidative stress and inflammation. *Nutrients.* 2024;16(4):507.

[114] Zhao B. Natural antioxidants protect neurons in Alzheimer's disease and Parkinson's disease. *Neurochemical Research.* 2009;34:630-8.

[115] Milkovic L, Siems W, Siems R, Zarkovic N. Oxidative stress and antioxidants in carcinogenesis and integrative therapy of cancer. *Current pharmaceutical design.* 2014;20(42):6529-42.

[116] Abbasi A, Saadat TR, Saadat YR. Microbial exopolysaccharides–β-glucans–as promising postbiotic candidates in vaccine adjuvants. *International Journal of Biological Macromolecules*. 2022;223:346-61.

[117] Gezginç Y, Karabekmez-erdem T, Tatar HD, Ayman S, Ganiyusufoğlu E, Dayısoylu KS. Health promoting benefits of postbiotics produced by lactic acid bacteria: Exopolysaccharide. *Biotech Studies.* 2022;31(2):61-70.

[118] Pourjafar H, Ansari F, Sadeghi A, Samakkhah SA, Jafari SM. Functional and health-promoting properties of probiotics' exopolysaccharides; isolation, characterization, and applications in the food industry. *Critical Reviews in Food Science and Nutrition.* 2023;63(26):8194-225.

[119] Yang S, Xu X, Peng Q, Ma L, Qiao Y, Shi B. Exopolysaccharides from lactic acid bacteria, as an alternative to antibiotics, on regulation of intestinal health and the immune system. *Animal Nutrition.* 2023;13:78-89.

[120] Xie Z, Bai Y, Chen G, Rui Y, Chen D, Sun Y, et al. Modulation of gut homeostasis by exopolysaccharides from Aspergillus cristatus (MK346334), a strain of fungus isolated from Fuzhuan brick tea, contributes to immunomodulatory activity in cyclophosphamide-treated mice. *Food & Function.* 2020;11(12):10397-412.

[121] Abbasi A, Kafil HS, Ozma MA, Sangtarash N, Sabahi S. Can food matrices be considered as a potential carrier for COVID-19? *Le infezioni in medicina.* 2022;30(1):59.

[122] Scarpellini E, Rinninella E, Basilico M, Colomier E, Rasetti C, Larussa T, et al. From pre-and probiotics to post-biotics: a narrative review. *International journal of environmental research and public health.* 2021;19(1):37.

[123] Petrosino S, Di Marzo V. The pharmacology of palmitoylethanolamide and first data on the therapeutic efficacy of some of its new formulations. *British journal of pharmacology.* 2017;174(11):1349-65.

[124] Laubach J, Joseph M, Brenza T, Gadhamshetty V, Sani RK. Exopolysaccharide and biopolymer-derived films as tools for transdermal drug delivery. *Journal of Controlled Release.* 2021;329:971-87.

[125] Sheikh T, Hamid B, Baba Z, Iqbal S, Yatoo A, Fatima S, et al. Extracellular polymeric substances in psychrophilic cyanobacteria: A potential bioflocculant and carbon sink to mitigate cold stress. *Biocatalysis and Agricultural Biotechnology.* 2022;42:102375.

[126] Okaiyeto K, Nwodo UU, Okoli SA, Mabinya LV, Okoh AI. Implications for public health demands alternatives to inorganic and synthetic flocculants: bioflocculants as important candidates. *MicrobiologyOpen.* 2016;5(2):177-211.

[127] Kiran NS, Yashaswini C, Singh S, Prajapati BG. Revisiting microbial exopolysaccharides: a biocompatible and sustainable polymeric material for multifaceted biomedical applications. *3 Biotech.* 2024;14(4):95.

[128] Zaghloul EH. Harnessing Lactic Acid Bacteria: A Pathway to Functional Food from Marine Seaweed. *Egyptian Journal of Aquatic Biology and Fisheries.* 2024;28(3):851-87.

[129] Gurunathan S, Thangaraj P, Kim JH. *Postbiotics-Functional Food Materials.* 2023.

[130] Aggarwal S, Sabharwal V, Kaushik P, Joshi A, Aayushi A, Suri M. Postbiotics: From emerging concept to application. *Frontiers in Sustainable Food Systems.* 2022;6:887642.

[131] Islam F, Azmat F, Imran A, Zippi M, Hong W, Tariq F, et al. Role of postbiotics in food and health: a comprehensive review. *CyTA-Journal of Food.* 2024;22(1):2386412.

[132] Rad AH, Abbasi A, Kafil HS, Ganbarov K. Potential pharmaceutical and food applications of postbiotics: a review. *Current pharmaceutical biotechnology.* 2020;21(15):1576-87.

[133] Wolf AJ, Underhill DM. Peptidoglycan *Nature Reviews Immunology.* recognition by the innate immune system. *Nature Reviews Immunology.* 2018;18(4):243-54.

[134] Santecchia I, Ferrer MF, Vieira ML, Gómez RM, Werts C. Phagocyte escape of Leptospira: the role of TLRs and NLRs. *Frontiers in immunology.* 2020;11:571816.

[135] Abouelela ME, Helmy YA. Next-generation probiotics as novel therapeutics for improving human health: current trends and future perspectives. *Microorganisms.* 2024;12(3):430.

[136] Tojo R, Suárez A, Clemente MG, de los Reyes-Gavilán CG, Margolles A, Gueimonde M, Ruas-Madiedo P. Intestinal microbiota in health and disease: role of bifidobacteria in gut homeostasis. *World journal of gastroenterology: WJG.* 2014;20(41):15163.

[137] Kucuksezer UC, Ozdemir C, Yazici D, Pat Y, Mitamura Y, Li M, et al. The epithelial barrier theory: development and exacerbation of allergic and other chronic inflammatory diseases. *Asia Pacific Allergy.* 2023;13(1):28-39.

[138] Liebregts T, Adam B, Bredack C, Röth A, Heinzel S, Lester S, et al. Immune activation in patients with irritable bowel syndrome. *Gastroenterology.* 2007;132(3):913-20.

[139] Chifiriuc MC, Holban AM, Curutiu C, Ditu L-M, Mihaescu G, Oprea AE, et al. Antibiotic drug delivery systems for the intracellular targeting of bacterial pathogens. *Smart drug delivery system: IntechOpen*; 2016.

[140] Thorakkattu P, Khanashyam AC, Shah K, Babu KS, Mundanat AS, Deliephan A, et al. Postbiotics: current trends in food and pharmaceutical industry. *Foods.* 2022;11(19):3094.

[141] Fritzsch FS, Dusny C, Frick O, Schmid A. Single-cell analysis in biotechnology, systems biology, and biocatalysis. *Annual review of chemical and biomolecular engineering.* 2012;3(1):129-55.

[142] Riwes M, Reddy P, editors. Short chain fatty acids: postbiotics/metabolites and graft versus host disease colitis. *Seminars in hematology;* 2020: Elsevier.

[143] Shi J, Wang Y, Cheng L, Wang J, Raghavan V. Gut microbiome modulation by probiotics, prebiotics, synbiotics and postbiotics: A novel strategy in food allergy prevention and treatment. *Critical Reviews in Food Science and Nutrition.* 2024;64(17):5984-6000.

[144] Blaak E, Canfora E, Theis S, Frost G, Groen A, Mithieux G, et al. Short chain fatty acids in human gut and metabolic health. *Beneficial microbes.* 2020;11(5):411-55.

[145] Russo E, Giudici F, Fiorindi C, Ficari F, Scaringi S, Amedei A. Immunomodulating activity and therapeutic effects of short chain fatty acids and tryptophan post-biotics in inflammatory bowel disease. *Frontiers in immunology.* 2019;10:2754.

[146] Yamashita JW. *Butyrate, Bacteriodes thetaiotaomicron and Campylobacter jejuni modulate the expression of beta-defensins, toll-like receptors and cytokines in Caco-2 cells:* University of Lethbridge (Canada); 2016.

[147] Silva YP, Bernardi A, Frozza RL. The role of short-chain fatty acids from gut microbiota in gut-brain communication. *Frontiers in endocrinology*. 2020;11:508738.
[148] Dicks LM. Gut bacteria and neurotransmitters. *Microorganisms*. 2022;10(9):1838.
[149] Janiad S, Rehman K. Microbiome-Targeted Therapies: Enhancing Resilience in Metabolic Disorders. *Human Microbiome: Techniques, Strategies, and Therapeutic Potential:* Springer; 2024. p. 401-36.
[150] Chambers ES, Morrison DJ, Frost G. Control of appetite and energy intake by SCFA: what are the potential underlying mechanisms? *Proceedings of the Nutrition Society*. 2015;74(3):328-36.
[151] Fu X, Liu Z, Zhu C, Mou H, Kong Q. Nondigestible carbohydrates, butyrate, and butyrate-producing bacteria. *Critical reviews in food science and nutrition*. 2019;59(sup1):S130-S52.
[152] Rivière A, Selak M, Lantin D, Leroy F, De Vuyst L. Bifidobacteria and butyrate-producing colon bacteria: importance and strategies for their stimulation in the human gut. *Frontiers in microbiology*. 2016;7:979.
[153] Jakubczyk D, Leszczyńska K, Górska S. The effectiveness of probiotics in the treatment of inflammatory bowel disease (IBD)—a critical review. *Nutrients*. 2020;12(7):1973.
[154] Zhuang X, Li T, Li M, Huang S, Qiu Y, Feng R, et al. Systematic review and meta-analysis: short-chain fatty acid characterization in patients with inflammatory bowel disease. *Inflammatory bowel diseases*. 2019;25(11):1751-63.
[155] Nowak A, Zakłos-Szyda M, Rosicka-Kaczmarek J, Motyl I. Anticancer potential of post-fermentation media and cell extracts of probiotic strains: an in vitro study. *Cancers*. 2022;14(7):1853.
[156] Czerucka D, Piche T, Rampal P. yeast as probiotics–Saccharomyces boulardii. *Alimentary pharmacology & therapeutics*. 2007;26(6):767-78.
[157] Colucci Cante R, Nigro F, Passannanti F, Lentini G, Gallo M, Nigro R, Budelli AL. Gut health benefits and associated systemic effects provided by functional components from the fermentation of natural matrices. *Comprehensive Reviews in Food Science and Food Safety*. 2024;23(3):e13356.
[158] Garcia F. Cell wall disruption and lysis. *Downstream Industrial Biotechnology: Recovery and Purification*. 2013:81-94.
[159] Grishin AV, Karyagina AS, Vasina DV, Vasina IV, Gushchin VA, Lunin VG. Resistance to peptidoglycan-degrading enzymes. *Critical Reviews in Microbiology*. 2020;46(6):703-26.
[160] de Azevedo Seara MFM. *Sustainable Production of Postbiotics for Food Applications:* Universidade Catolica Portuguesa (Portugal); 2023.
[161] Peluzio MdCG, Martinez JA, Milagro FI. Postbiotics: Metabolites and mechanisms involved in microbiota-host interactions. *Trends in Food Science & Technology*. 2021;108:11-26.
[162] Tan SN, Yong JWH, Teo CC, Ge L, Chan YW, Hew CS. Determination of metabolites in Uncaria sinensis by HPLC and GC–MS after green solvent microwave-assisted extraction. *Talanta*. 2011;83(3):891-8.

[163] Al-Habsi N, Al-Khalili M, Haque SA, Elias M, Olqi NA, Al Uraimi T. Health Benefits of Prebiotics, Probiotics, Synbiotics, and Postbiotics. *Nutrients.* 2024;16(22):3955.

[164] Li H-Y, Zhou D-D, Gan R-Y, Huang S-Y, Zhao C-N, Shang A, et al. Effects and mechanisms of probiotics, prebiotics, synbiotics, and postbiotics on metabolic diseases targeting gut microbiota: A narrative review. *Nutrients.* 2021;13(9):3211.

[165] Gupta D, Lall A, Kumar S, Patil TD, Gaikwad KK. Plant based edible films and coatings for food packaging applications: Recent advances, applications, and trends. *Sustainable Food Technology*. 2024.

[166] Nataraj BH, Ali SA, Behare PV, Yadav H. Postbiotics-parabiotics: The new horizons in microbial biotherapy and functional foods. *Microbial cell factories.* 2020;19:1-22.

[167] Moradi M, Kousheh SA, Almasi H, Alizadeh A, Guimarães JT, Yılmaz N, Lotfi A. Postbiotics produced by lactic acid bacteria: The next frontier in food safety. *Comprehensive reviews in food science and food safety*. 2020;19(6):3390-415.

[168] McKeen L. Introduction to food irradiation and medical sterilization. *The Effect of sterilization on plastics and elastomers.* 2012:1.

[169] Jastrząb R, Tomecki R, Jurkiewicz A, Graczyk D, Szczepankowska AK, Mytych J, et al. The strain-dependent cytostatic activity of Lactococcus lactis on CRC cell lines is mediated through the release of arginine deiminase. *Microbial Cell Factories.* 2024;23(1):82.

[170] Moy FJ, Haraki K, Mobilio D, Walker G, Powers R, Tabei K, et al. MS/NMR: a structure-based approach for discovering protein ligands and for drug design by coupling size exclusion chromatography, mass spectrometry, and nuclear magnetic resonance spectroscopy. *Analytical chemistry*. 2001;73(3):571-81.

[171] El Far MS, Zakaria AS, Kassem MA, Wedn A, Guimei M, Edward EA. Promising biotherapeutic prospects of different probiotics and their derived postbiotic metabolites: in-vitro and histopathological investigation. *BMC microbiology*. 2023;23(1):122.

[172] Liu C, Ma N, Feng Y, Zhou M, Li H, Zhang X, Ma X. From probiotics to postbiotics: Concepts and applications. *Animal Research and One Health.* 2023;1(1):92-114.

[173] de Almeida Godoy CL, Costa LM, Guerra CA, de Oliveira VS, de Paula BP, Lemos Junior WJF, et al. Potentially postbiotic-containing preservative to extend the use-by date of raw chicken sausages and semifinished chicken products. *Sustainability*. 2022;14(5):2646.

[174] Pyo Y, Kwon KH, Jung YJ. Probiotic functions in fermented foods: anti-viral, immunomodulatory, and anti-cancer benefits. *Foods.* 2024;13(15):2386.

[175] Mahooti M, Abdolalipour E, Sanami S, Zare D. Inflammatory Modulation Effects of Probiotics: A Safe and Promising Modulator for Cancer Prevention. *Current microbiology*. 2024;81(11):372.

[176] Rad AH, Aghebati-Maleki L, Kafil HS, Abbasi A. Molecular mechanisms of postbiotics in colorectal cancer prevention and treatment. *Critical reviews in food science and nutrition.* 2021;61(11):1787-803.

[177] Wang R, Yu Y, Yu W, Sun S, Lei Y, Li Y, et al. Roles of Probiotics, Prebiotics, and Postbiotics in B-cell mediated Immune Regulation. *The Journal of Nutrition.* 2024.

[178] Chandra P, Sharma H, Sachan N. The Potential Role of Prebiotics, Probiotics, and Synbiotics in Cancer Prevention and Therapy. *Synbiotics in Metabolic Disorders.* 191-213.

[179] Blazheva D, Mihaylova D, Averina O, Slavchev A, Brazkova M, Poluektova E, et al. Antioxidant potential of probiotics and postbiotics: a biotechnological approach to improving their stability. *Russian Journal of Genetics.* 2022;58(9):1036-50.

[180] Teame T, Wang A, Xie M, Zhang Z, Yang Y, Ding Q, et al. Paraprobiotics and postbiotics of probiotic Lactobacilli, their positive effects on the host and action mechanisms: A review. *Frontiers in nutrition.* 2020;7:570344.

[181] Elhawary EA, Korany DA, Eldahshan OA, Singab ANB. *Insights on Dietary Anticancer Products: Food Supplements, Prebiotics, and Probiotics*. Springer; 2024.

[182] Park M, Joung M, Park J-H, Ha SK, Park H-Y. Role of postbiotics in diet-induced metabolic disorders. *Nutrients.* 2022;14(18):3701.

[183] Natesan V, Kim S-J. Lipid metabolism, disorders and therapeutic drugs–review. *Biomolecules & therapeutics*. 2021;29(6):596.

[184] Das S, Mohan V. *Disorders of lipid metabolism. API text Book of medicine, 75th edition association of physician of India,* Mumbai. 2003:250-8.

[185] Ma J, Piao X, Mahfuz S, Long S, Wang J. The interaction among gut microbes, the intestinal barrier and short chain fatty acids. *Animal Nutrition*. 2022;9:159-74.

[186] Park S-J, Sharma A, Lee H-J. Postbiotics against obesity: perception and overview based on pre-clinical and clinical studies. International Journal of Molecular Sciences. 2023;24(7):6414.

[187] Liu Y, Wang J, Wu C. Modulation of gut microbiota and immune system by probiotics, pre-biotics, and post-biotics. *Frontiers in nutrition.* 2022;8:634897.

[188] Mak KM, Shekhar AC. Lipopolysaccharide, arbiter of the gut–liver axis, modulates hepatic cell pathophysiology in alcoholism. *The Anatomical Record.* 2024.

[189] Khani N, Noorkhajavi G, Reziabad RH, Rad AH, Ziavand M. Postbiotics as potential detoxification tools for mitigation of pesticides. *Probiotics and Antimicrobial Proteins.* 2024;16(4):1427-39.

[190] Shokatayeva D, Savitskaya I, Kistaubayeva A, editors. *Wound-healing activity of immobilized postbiotics from Bacillus subtilis exometabolites*. BIO Web of Conferences; 2021: EDP Sciences.

[191] Zamanpour S, Noori SMA, Yancheshmeh BS, Afshari A, Hashemi M. A systematic review to introduce the most effective postbiotics derived from probiotics for aflatoxin detoxification in vitro. *Italian Journal of Food Science.* 2023;35(4):31-49.

[192] Jani RK. Gastrointestinal Tract and Digestion Challenges in Chronic Diseases and Applications of Functional Foods and Nutraceuticals. *Molecular Mechanisms of*

Action of Functional Foods and Nutraceuticals for Chronic Diseases: CRC Press; 2023. p. 307-64.

[193] Panpetch W, Phuengmaung P, Cheibchalard T, Somboonna N, Leelahavanichkul A, Tumwasorn S. Lacticaseibacillus casei strain T21 attenuates Clostridioides difficile infection in a murine model through reduction of inflammation and gut dysbiosis with decreased toxin lethality and enhanced mucin production. *Frontiers in microbiology*. 2021;12:745299.

[194] Kaistha SD, Deshpande N. Traditional probiotics, next-generation probiotics and engineered live biotherapeutic products in chronic wound healing. *Wound Healing Research: Current Trends and Future Directions*. 2021:247-84.

[195] Shopova D, Mihaylova A, Yaneva A, Bakova D, Dimova-Gabrovska M. Biofabrication Approaches for Peri-Implantitis Tissue Regeneration: A Focus on Bioprinting Methods. *Prosthesis*. 2024;6(2):372-92.

[196] Heo YM, Lee D-G, Mun S, Kim M, Baek C, Lee H, et al. Skin benefits of postbiotics derived from Micrococcus luteus derived from human skin: an untapped potential for dermatological health. *Genes & Genomics*. 2024;46(1):13-25.

[197] Mihai MM, Bălăceanu-Gurău B, Ion A, Holban AM, Gurău C-D, Popescu MN, et al. Host–Microbiome Crosstalk in Chronic Wound Healing. *International Journal of Molecular Sciences*. 2024;25(9):4629.

[198] Szydłowska A, Sionek B. Probiotics and postbiotics as the functional food components affecting the immune response. *Microorganisms*. 2022;11(1):104.

[199] Sadeghi A, Ebrahimi M, Shahryari S, Kharazmi MS, Jafari SM. Food applications of probiotic yeasts; focusing on their techno-functional, postbiotic and protective capabilities. *Trends in Food Science & Technology. 2022*;128:278-95.

[200] Kapustian A, Cherno N, Naumenko K, Gural L, Osolina S. Regulation of Functional Foods in Ukraine and the World. Prospects for the Use of Postbiotics as Functional Ingredients. *Food Science & Technology* (2073-8684). 2023;17(2).

[201] Fernández J, Redondo-Blanco S, Gutiérrez-del-Río I, Miguélez EM, Villar CJ, Lombo F. Colon microbiota fermentation of dietary prebiotics towards short-chain fatty acids and their roles as anti-inflammatory and antitumour agents: A review. *Journal of Functional Foods*. 2016;25:511-22.

[202] Hanaway P. Balance of floral, galt, and mucosal integrity. *Alternative Therapies in Health & Medicine*. 2006;12(5).

[203] Mirmiran P, Bahadoran Z, Azizi F. Functional foods-based diet as a novel dietary approach for management of type 2 diabetes and its complications: A review. *World journal of diabetes*. 2014;5(3):267.

[204] Balthazar CF, Guimarães JF, Coutinho NM, Pimentel TC, Ranadheera CS, Santillo A, et al. The future of functional food: Emerging technologies application on prebiotics, probiotics and postbiotics. *Comprehensive Reviews in Food Science and Food Safety*. 2022;21(3):2560-86.

[205] Kouhounde S, Adéoti K, Mounir M, Giusti A, Refinetti P, Otu A, et al. Applications of probiotic-based multi-components to human, animal and ecosystem health: concepts, methodologies, and action mechanisms. *Microorganisms*. 2022;10(9):1700.

[206] Wang K, Zhao X, Yang S, Qi X, Li A, Yu W. New insights into dairy management and the prevention and treatment of osteoporosis: The shift from single nutrient to dairy matrix effects—A review. *Comprehensive Reviews in Food Science and Food Safety*. 2024;23(4):e13374.

[207] Summer M, Sajjad A, Ali S, Hussain T. Exploring the underlying correlation between microbiota, immune system, hormones, and inflammation with breast cancer and the role of probiotics, prebiotics and postbiotics. *Archives of Microbiology*. 2024;206(4):145.

[208] Salminen S, Collado MC, Endo A, Hill C, Lebeer S, Quigley EM, et al. The International Scientific Association of Probiotics and Prebiotics (ISAPP) consensus statement on the definition and scope of postbiotics. *Nature Reviews Gastroenterology & Hepatology*. 2021;18(9):649-67.

[209] Abbasi A, Sheykhsaran E, Kafil HS. *Postbiotics: science, technology and applications:* Bentham Science Publishers; 2021.

[210] İncili GK, Karatepe P, Akgöl M, Güngören A, Koluman A, İlhak Oİ, et al. Characterization of lactic acid bacteria postbiotics, evaluation in-vitro antibacterial effect, microbial and chemical quality on chicken drumsticks. *Food Microbiology*. 2022;104:104001.

[211] Abbasi A, Hashemi M, Pourjafar H, Hosseini SM, Kafil HS, Rad AH, et al. Chemical Characterization, Cell-Based Safety, and Antioxidant Assessments of Lactobacillus helveticus Postbiotics and Their Potential Antibacterial Effects and Mode of Action Against Food-Borne Multidrug-Resistant Staphylococcus aureus and Enterohaemorrhagic Escherichia coli O157: H7. *Journal of Food Safety*. 2024;44(6):e13174.

[212] Ozma MA, Hosseini HM, Ataee MH, Mirhosseini SA. Evaluating the antibacterial, antibiofilm, and anti-toxigenic effects of postbiotics from lactic acid bacteria on Clostridium difficile. *Iranian Journal of Microbiology*. 2024;16(4):497-508.

[213] Ozma MA, Khodadadi E, Pakdel F, Kamounah FS, Yousefi M, Yousefi B, et al. Baicalin, a natural antimicrobial and anti-biofilm agent. *Journal of Herbal Medicine*. 2021;27:100432.

[214] Ozma MA, Ghotaslou R, Asgharzadeh M, Abbasi A, Rezaee MA, Kafil HS. Cytotoxicity assessment and antimicrobial effects of cell-free supernatants from probiotic lactic acid bacteria and yeast against multi-drug resistant Escherichia coli. *Letters in Applied Microbiology*. 2024;77(9):ovae084.

[215] Ozma MA, Alileh NF, Abbasi A, Mahdavi S, Fadaee M, Nezhadi J, et al. Antibacterial, antibiofilm, and gene expression assessment of Ajwain (Trachyspermum ammi) essential oil on drug-resistant gastrointestinal pathogens and its combination effect with ampicillin. *Letters in Applied Microbiology*. 2024:ovae138.

[216] Ozma MA, Maroufi P, Khodadadi E, Köse Ş, Esposito I, Ganbarov K, et al. Clinical manifestation, diagnosis, prevention and control of SARS-CoV-2 (COVID-19) during the outbreak period. *Infez Med*. 2020;28(2):153-65.

[217] Ozma MA, Abbasi A, Akrami S, Lahouty M, Shahbazi N, Ganbarov K, et al. Postbiotics as the key mediators of the gut microbiota-host interactions. *Le infezioni in medicina.* 2022;30(2):180.

[218] Asghari Ozma M, Lahouty M, Fallahi Alileh N, Mahdavi S, Asghari Ozma M, Nezhadi J, et al. Application of Proteomics in Medical Bacteriology with Emphasis on Proteomic Analysis of Postbiotics. *Medical Journal of Mashhad University of Medical Sciences.* 2024;67(3).

[219] Ozma MA, Fadaee M, Hosseini HM, Ataee MH, Mirhosseini SA. A Critical Review of Postbiotics as Promising Novel Therapeutic Agents for Clostridial Infections. *Probiotics and Antimicrobial Proteins.* 2024:1-12.

[220] Boahen A, Than LTL, Loke Y-L, Chew SY. The antibiofilm role of biotics Family in vaginal fungal infections. *Frontiers in Microbiology.* 2022;13:787119.

[221] Machado A, Zamora-Mendoza L, Alexis F, Álvarez-Suarez JM. Use of plant extracts, bee-derived products, and probiotic-related applications to fight multidrug-resistant pathogens in the post-antibiotic era. *Future Pharmacology.* 2023;3(3):535-67.

[222] Abbasi A, Rad AH, Ghasempour Z, Sabahi S, Kafil HS, Hasannezhad P, et al. The biological activities of postbiotics in gastrointestinal disorders. *Critical Reviews in Food Science and Nutrition.* 2022;62(22):5983-6004.

[223] Ozma MA, Khodadadi E, Rezaee MA, Kamounah FS, Asgharzadeh M, Ganbarov K, et al. Induction of proteome changes involved in biofilm formation of Enterococcus faecalis in response to gentamicin. *Microbial Pathogenesis.* 2021;157:105003.

[224] Ozma MA, Lahouty M, Abbasi A, Rezaee MA, Kafil HS, Asgharzadeh M. Effective bacterial factors involved in the dissemination of tuberculosis. *Biointerface Res Appl Chem.* 2022;13:234.

[225] Asgharzadeh M, Ozma MA, Rashedi J, Poor BM, Agharzadeh V, Vegari A, et al. False-positive Mycobacterium tuberculosis detection: Ways to prevent cross-contamination. *Tuberculosis and Respiratory Diseases.* 2020;83(3):211.

[226] Liu Y, Wang J, Wu C. Microbiota and tuberculosis: a potential role of probiotics, and postbiotics. *Frontiers in Nutrition.* 2021;8:626254.

[227] Ozma MA, Rashedi J, Poor BM, Vegari A, Asgharzadeh V, Kafil HS, et al. Tuberculosis and diabetes mellitus in Northwest of Iran. *Infectious Disorders-Drug Targets (Formerly Current Drug Targets-Infectious Disorders).* 2020;20(5):667-71.

[228] Asgharzadeh V, Rezaei SAS, Asgharzadeh M, Rashedi J, Kafil HS, Nobari HJ, et al. Host Risk Factors for Tuberculosis. *Infectious disorders drug targets.*

[229] Mantziari A, Salminen S, Szajewska H, Malagón-Rojas JN. Postbiotics against pathogens commonly involved in pediatric infectious diseases. *Microorganisms.* 2020;8(10):1510.

[230] Rawal S, Ali SA. Probiotics and postbiotics play a role in maintaining dermal health. *Food & Function.* 2023;14(9):3966-81.

[231] Zavišić G, Ristić S, Petričević S, Janković D, Petković B. Microbial Contamination of Food: Probiotics and Postbiotics as Potential Biopreservatives. *Foods.* 2024;13(16):2487.

[232] Ozma MA, Abbasi A, Asgharzadeh M, Pagliano P, Guarino A, Köse Ş, Kafil HS. Antibiotic therapy for pan-drug-resistant infections. *Le infezioni in medicina.* 2022;30(4):525.

[233] Favero C, Giordano L, Mihaila SM, Masereeuw R, Ortiz A, Sanchez-Niño MD. Postbiotics and kidney disease. *Toxins.* 2022;14(9):623.

[234] Watson RA. Enlisting probiotics to combat recurrent urinary tract infections in women—A military strategy for meeting the challenge. *Antibiotics.* 2023;12(1):167.

[235] Van VTH, Liu Z-S, Hsieh Y-J, Shiu W-C, Chen B-Y, Ku Y-W, Chen P-W. Therapeutic effects of orally administration of viable and inactivated probiotic strains against murine urinary tract infection. *Journal of Food and Drug Analysis.* 2023;31(4):583.

[236] Reid G, Bruce AW. Probiotics to prevent urinary tract infections: the rationale and evidence. *World journal of urology.* 2006;24:28-32.

[237] Ng QX, Peters C, Venkatanarayanan N, Goh YY, Ho CYX, Yeo W-S. Use of Lactobacillus spp. to prevent recurrent urinary tract infections in females. *Medical hypotheses.* 2018;114:49-54.

[238] de Llano DG, Arroyo A, Cárdenas N, Rodríguez JM, Moreno-Arribas MV, Bartolomé B. Strain-specific inhibition of the adherence of uropathogenic bacteria to bladder cells by probiotic Lactobacillus spp. *Pathogens and disease.* 2017;75(4):ftx043.

[239] Fusco A, Savio V, Chiaromonte A, Alfano A, D'Ambrosio S, Cimini D, Donnarumma G. Evaluation of Different Activity of Lactobacillus spp. against Two Proteus mirabilis Isolated Clinical Strains in Different Anatomical Sites In Vitro: An Explorative Study to Improve the Therapeutic Approach. *Microorganisms.* 2023;11(9):2201.

[240] De Gregorio PR, Tomás MSJ, Terraf MCL, Nader-Macías MEF. In vitro and in vivo effects of beneficial vaginal lactobacilli on pathogens responsible for urogenital tract infections. *Journal of medical microbiology.* 2014;63(5):685-96.

[241] Darouiche RO, Hull RA. Bacterial interference for prevention of urinary tract infection. *Clinical infectious diseases.* 2012;55(10):1400-7.

[242] Shazadi K, Arshad N. Evaluation of inhibitory and probiotic properties of lactic acid bacteria isolated from vaginal microflora. *Folia Microbiologica.* 2022;67(3):427-45.

[243] Malagón-Rojas JN, Mantziari A, Salminen S, Szajewska H. Postbiotics for preventing and treating common infectious diseases in children: a systematic review. *Nutrients.* 2020;12(2):389.

[244] Mindt BC, DiGiandomenico A. Microbiome modulation as a novel strategy to treat and prevent respiratory infections. *Antibiotics.* 2022;11(4):474.

[245] Ozma MA, Khodadadi E, Rezaee MA, Asgharzadeh M, Aghazadeh M, Zeinalzadeh E, et al. Bacterial proteomics and its application in pathogenesis studies. *Current pharmaceutical biotechnology.* 2022;23(10):1245-56.

[246] Ozma MA, Nabizadeh E, Valiollahzadeh MR, Rashedi J, Poor BM, Asgharzadeh V, et al. *Different Dimensions of the Effects of SARS-CoV-2 in Causing Fluctuations in the Blood Pressure of Patients.* 2022.

[247] Andrade JC, Kumar S, Kumar A, Černáková L, Rodrigues CF. Application of probiotics in candidiasis management. *Critical reviews in food science and nutrition.* 2022;62(30):8249-64.

[248] Rather IA, Choi S-B, Kamli MR, Hakeem KR, Sabir JS, Park Y-H, Hor Y-Y. Potential adjuvant therapeutic effect of Lactobacillus plantarum probio-88 postbiotics against SARS-COV-2. *Vaccines.* 2021;9(10):1067.

[249] Akatsu H. Exploring the effect of probiotics, prebiotics, and postbiotics in strengthening immune activity in the elderly. *Vaccines.* 2021;9(2):136.

[250] Humam AM, Loh TC, Foo HL, Izuddin WI, Zulkifli I, Samsudin AA, Mustapha NM. Supplementation of postbiotic RI11 improves antioxidant enzyme activity, upregulated gut barrier genes, and reduced cytokine, acute phase protein, and heat shock protein 70 gene expression levels in heat-stressed broilers. *Poultry science.* 2021;100(3):100908.

[251] Danilenko V, Devyatkin A, Marsova M, Shibilova M, Ilyasov R, Shmyrev V. Common inflammatory mechanisms in COVID-19 and Parkinson's diseases: The role of microbiome, pharmabiotics and postbiotics in their prevention. *Journal of Inflammation Research.* 2021:6349-81.

[252] Santiago-López L, Almada-Corral A, García HS, Mata-Haro V, González-Córdova AF, Vallejo-Cordoba B, Hernández-Mendoza A. Antidepressant and anxiolytic effects of fermented huauzontle, a Prehispanic Mexican pseudocereal. *Foods.* 2022;12(1):53.

[253] Diez-Martin E, Hernandez-Suarez L, Muñoz-Villafranca C, Martin-Souto L, Astigarraga E, Ramirez-Garcia A, Barreda-Gómez G. Inflammatory Bowel Disease: A Comprehensive Analysis of Molecular Bases, Predictive Biomarkers, Diagnostic Methods, and Therapeutic Options. *International Journal of Molecular Sciences.* 2024;25(13):7062.

[254] Dwivedi M, Kumar P, Laddha NC, Kemp EH. Induction of regulatory T cells: a role for probiotics and prebiotics to suppress autoimmunity. *Autoimmunity Reviews.* 2016;15(4):379-92.

[255] da Silva Vale A, de Melo Pereira GV, de Oliveira AC, de Carvalho Neto DP, Herrmann LW, Karp SG, et al. Production, formulation, and application of postbiotics in the treatment of skin conditions. *Fermentation.* 2023;9(3):264.

[256] De Almeida CV, Antiga E, Lulli M. Oral and topical probiotics and postbiotics in skincare and dermatological therapy: A concise review. *Microorganisms.* 2023;11(6):1420.

[257] Coppola S, Avagliano C, Sacchi A, Laneri S, Calignano A, Voto L, et al. Potential clinical applications of the postbiotic butyrate in human skin diseases. *Molecules.* 2022;27(6):1849.

[258] Wu Y, Wang Y, Hu A, Shu X, Huang W, Liu J, et al. Lactobacillus plantarum-derived postbiotics prevent Salmonella-induced neurological dysfunctions by modulating gut–brain axis in mice. *Frontiers in Nutrition.* 2022;9:946096.

[259] Głowacka P, Oszajca K, Pudlarz A, Szemraj J, Witusik-Perkowska M. Postbiotics as Molecules Targeting Cellular Events of Aging Brain—The Role in Pathogenesis, Prophylaxis and Treatment of Neurodegenerative Diseases. *Nutrients.* 2024;16(14):2244.

[260] Srivastava P, Kim K-s. Membrane vesicles derived from gut microbiota and probiotics: Cutting-edge therapeutic approaches for multidrug-resistant superbugs linked to neurological anomalies. *Pharmaceutics.* 2022;14(11):2370.

[261] Bulacios GA, Cataldo PG, Naja JR, de Chaves EP, Taranto MP, Minahk CJ, et al. Improvement of Key Molecular Events Linked to Alzheimer's Disease Pathology Using Postbiotics. *ACS omega.* 2023;8(50):48042-9.

[262] Heniedy AM, Mahdy DM, Elenien WIA, Mourad S, El-Kadi RA. Postbiotics as a Health-Promoting Technique: A Review Article on Scientific and Commercial Interest. *Process Biochemistry.* 2024.

[263] Chan MZA, Liu S-Q. Fortifying foods with synbiotic and postbiotic preparations of the probiotic yeast, Saccharomyces boulardii. *Current Opinion in Food Science.* 2022;43:216-24.

[264] Bermudez-Brito M, Plaza-Díaz J, Muñoz-Quezada S, Gómez-Llorente C, Gil A. Probiotic mechanisms of action. *Annals of Nutrition and Metabolism.* 2012;61(2):160-74.

[265] Plaza-Diaz J, Ruiz-Ojeda FJ, Gil-Campos M, Gil A. Mechanisms of action of probiotics. *Advances in nutrition.* 2019;10:S49-S66.

[266] Wang G, Ding T, Ai L. Effects and mechanisms of probiotics, prebiotics, synbiotics and postbiotics on intestinal health and disease. *Frontiers Media SA;* 2024. p. 1430312.

[267] Gao J, Li Y, Wan Y, Hu T, Liu L, Yang S, et al. A novel postbiotic from Lactobacillus rhamnosus GG with a beneficial effect on intestinal barrier function. *Frontiers in microbiology.* 2019;10:477.

[268] Parhi P. Relationship Between Antimicrobial Peptides, Probiotics, Postbiotics. *Evolution of Antimicrobial Peptides: From Self-Defense to Therapeutic Applications.* 199.

[269] Krsek A, Baticic L. Neutrophils in the Focus: Impact on Neuroimmune Dynamics and the Gut–Brain Axis. *Gastrointestinal Disorders.* 2024;6(3):557-606.

[270] Kandpal M, Indari O, Baral B, Jakhmola S, Tiwari D, Bhandari V, et al. Dysbiosis of Gut Microbiota from the Perspective of the Gut–Brain Axis: Role in the Provocation of Neurological Disorders. *Metabolites.* 2022;12(11):1064.

[271] Holzer P, Farzi A, Hassan AM, Zenz G, Jačan A, Reichmann F. Visceral inflammation and immune activation stress the brain. *Frontiers in immunology.* 2017;8:1613.

[272] Pothuraju R, Chaudhary S, Rachagani S, Kaur S, Roy HK, Bouvet M, Batra SK. Mucins, gut microbiota, and postbiotics role in colorectal cancer. *Gut microbes.* 2021;13(1):1974795.

[273] Jastrząb R, Graczyk D, Siedlecki P. Molecular and cellular mechanisms influenced by postbiotics. *International journal of molecular sciences.* 2021;22(24):13475.

[274] Salva S, Tiscornia I, Gutiérrez F, Alvarez S, Bollati-Fogolín M. Lactobacillus rhamnosus postbiotic-induced immunomodulation as safer alternative to the use of live bacteria. *Cytokine.* 2021;146:155631.

[275] Yan R, Zeng X, Shen J, Wu Z, Guo Y, Du Q, et al. New clues for postbiotics to improve host health: a review from the perspective of function and mechanisms. *Journal of the Science of Food and Agriculture.* 2024.

[276] Vinderola G, Sanders ME, Salminen S. The concept of postbiotics. *Foods.* 2022;11(8):1077.

[277] Gasaly N, De Vos P, Hermoso MA. Impact of bacterial metabolites on gut barrier function and host immunity: a focus on bacterial metabolism and its relevance for intestinal inflammation. *Frontiers in immunology.* 2021;12:658354.

[278] Mohseni AH, Casolaro V, Bermúdez-Humarán LG, Keyvani H, Taghinezhad-S S. Modulation of the PI3K/Akt/mTOR signaling pathway by probiotics as a fruitful target for orchestrating the immune response. *Gut Microbes.* 2021;13(1):1886844.

[279] De Vos WM, Tilg H, Van Hul M, Cani PD. Gut microbiome and health: mechanistic insights. *Gut.* 2022;71(5):1020-32.

[280] Bach Knudsen KE, Lærke HN, Hedemann MS, Nielsen TS, Ingerslev AK, Gundelund Nielsen DS, et al. Impact of diet-modulated butyrate production on intestinal barrier function and inflammation. *Nutrients.* 2018;10(10):1499.

[281] Llewellyn A, Foey A. Probiotic modulation of innate cell pathogen sensing and signaling events. *Nutrients.* 2017;9(10):1156.

[282] O'Riordan KJ, Collins MK, Moloney GM, Knox EG, Aburto MR, Fülling C, et al. Short chain fatty acids: microbial metabolites for gut-brain axis signalling. *Molecular and Cellular Endocrinology.* 2022;546:111572.

[283] Fang H, Rodrigues e-Lacerda R, Barra NG, Kukje Zada D, Robin N, Mehra A, Schertzer JD. Postbiotic impact on host metabolism and immunity provides therapeutic potential in metabolic disease. *Endocrine Reviews.* 2024:bnae025.

[284] Huang Z, Mu C, Chen Y, Zhu Z, Chen C, Lan L, et al. Effects of dietary probiotic supplementation on LXRα and CYP7α1 gene expression, liver enzyme activities and fat metabolism in ducks. *British poultry science.* 2015;56(2):218-24.

[285] Yang M, Zhang C-Y. G protein-coupled receptors as potential targets for nonalcoholic fatty liver disease treatment. *World Journal of Gastroenterology.* 2021;27(8):677.

[286] Chen J, Thomsen M, Vitetta L. Interaction of gut microbiota with dysregulation of bile acids in the pathogenesis of nonalcoholic fatty liver disease and potential therapeutic implications of probiotics. *Journal of cellular biochemistry.* 2019;120(3):2713-20.

[287] Fiorucci S, Cipriani S, Baldelli F, Mencarelli A. Bile acid-activated receptors in the treatment of dyslipidemia and related disorders. *Progress in lipid research.* 2010;49(2):171-85.

[288] Sellge G, Kufer TA, editors. PRR-signaling pathways: learning from microbial tactics. *Seminars in immunology;* 2015: Elsevier.

[289] Lu J, Shataer D, Yan H, Dong X, Zhang M, Qin Y, et al. Probiotics and Non-Alcoholic Fatty Liver Disease: Unveiling the Mechanisms of Lactobacillus plantarum and Bifidobacterium bifidum in Modulating Lipid Metabolism, Inflammation, and Intestinal Barrier Integrity. *Foods.* 2024;13(18):2992.

[290] Hu Q, Zhang W, Wu Z, Tian X, Xiang J, Li L, et al. Baicalin and the liver-gut system: Pharmacological bases explaining its therapeutic effects. *Pharmacological research.* 2021;165:105444.

[291] Wang Z, Chen W-D, Wang Y-D. Nuclear receptors: a bridge linking the gut microbiome and the host. *Molecular Medicine.* 2021;27(1):144.

[292] Kang G, Wang X, Gao M, Wang L, Feng Z, Meng S, et al. Propionate-producing engineered probiotics ameliorated murine ulcerative colitis by restoring anti-inflammatory macrophage via the GPR43/HDAC1/IL-10 axis. *Bioengineering & Translational Medicine.* 2024:e10682.

[293] Yiu JH, Dorweiler B, Woo CW. Interaction between gut microbiota and toll-like receptor: from immunity to metabolism. *Journal of Molecular Medicine.* 2017;95(1):13-20.

[294] Plaza-Diaz J, Gomez-Llorente C, Fontana L, Gil A. Modulation of immunity and inflammatory gene expression in the gut, in inflammatory diseases of the gut and in the liver by probiotics. *World journal of gastroenterology: WJG.* 2014;20(42):15632.

[295] Chen D, Jin D, Huang S, Wu J, Xu M, Liu T, et al. Clostridium butyricum, a butyrate-producing probiotic, inhibits intestinal tumor development through modulating Wnt signaling and gut microbiota. *Cancer letters.* 2020;469:456-67.

About the Authors

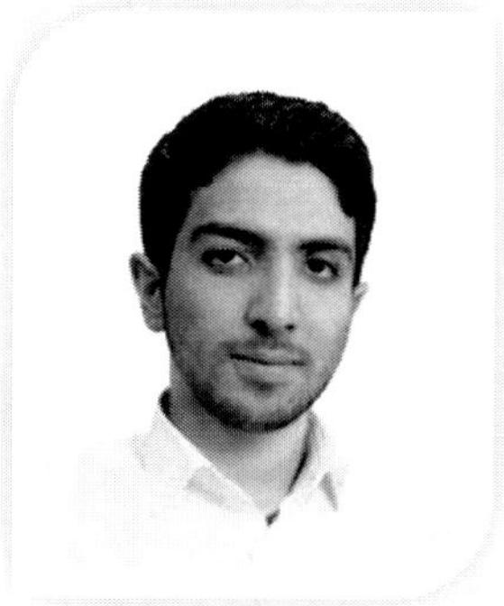

Mahdi Asghari Ozma
Department of Microbiology,
Tabriz University of Medical Sciences, Tabriz, Iran
Emails: asghariozma@tbzmed.ac.ir; asghariozma@gmail.com

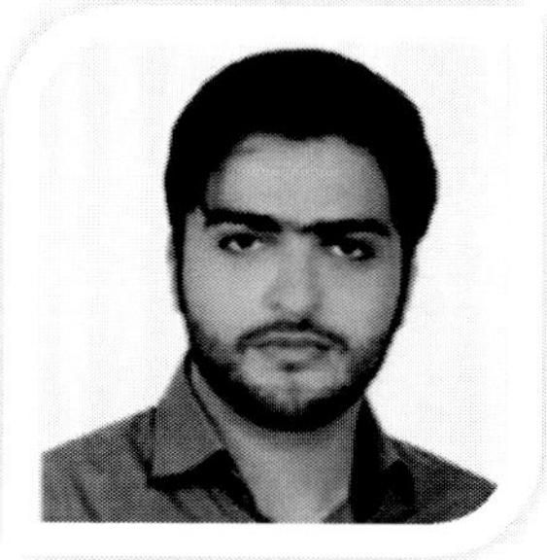

Amin Abbasi
Department of Food Science and Technology,
National Nutrition and Food Technology Research Institute,
Faculty of Nutrition Science and Food Technology, Shahid Beheshti University of Medical Sciences, Tehran, Iran
Emails: abbasia@sbmu.ac.ir; aminabasi.tbz.med.ac@gmail.com

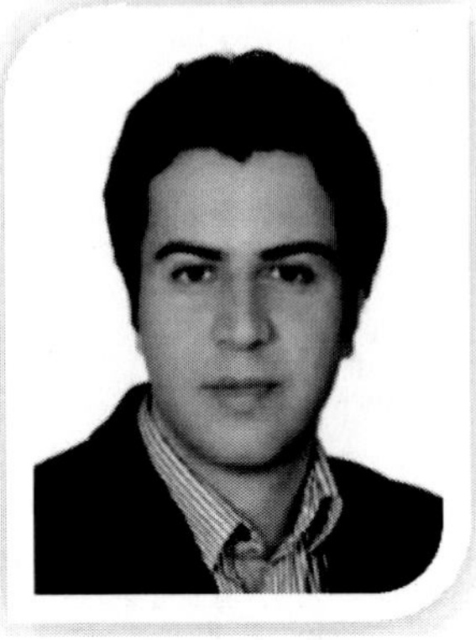

Hossein Samadi Kafil
Drug Applied Research Center,
Tabriz University of Medical Sciences, Tabriz, Iran
Emails: kafilhs@tbzmed.ac.ir; h.s.kafil@gmail.com

Index

F

G

H

I